AFTER THE FIGHT

AFTER THE FIGHT
Using Your Disagreements to Build a Stronger Relationship

DANIEL B. WILE

THE GUILFORD PRESS
New York   London

Library of Congress Cataloging-in-Publication Data

Wile, Daniel B.
    After the fight: a night in the life of a couple / Daniel B. Wile.
        p.   cm.
    Includes bibliographical references (p. 319) and index.
    ISBN 0-89862-754-0   ISBN 1-57230-026-4 (pbk.)
    1. Marital psychotherapy—Case studies. 2. Communication in marriage—Case studies. I. Title.
    RC488.5.W549 1993
    616.89'156—dc 20   93-4846
                                                      CIP

To Joanne R. Wile,
my favorite sparring partner.

Acknowledgments

This book emerged out of weekly meetings over 20 years with Bernard Apfelbaum, my mentor in ego analysis.

The book emerged in a more personal way out of my 27-year relationship with Joanne R. Wile.

Carol Carr breathed life into the book. She enriched the language, tightened the reasoning, smoothed the flow of words, and added a colloquial touch to the dialogues.

Nan Narboe helped straighten out my thinking and wording at several crucial points.

Philip A. Cowan showed me where the words and ideas flowed and where they stumbled, wandered, and sat on the page doing nothing.

Eleanor Bulova suggested better ways to include the couple's children and kept me consistent with my own approach.

Elaine K. Breshgold showed me connections (among various parts of the book) that I hadn't known were there.

Diana Weinstock showed me points where readers were likely to object or misunderstand.

Carolyn Pape Cowan enabled me to correct biases that I hadn't known were there.

Martin H. Williams helped me modify the overall tone of the book.

Geoffrey D. White identified points at which the book failed to address the concerns of contemporary psychotherapists.

Paul L. Wachtel pointed out what was new in what I was writing and helped me develop it a step further.

Howard P. Wile reviewed the final draft and corrected errors the rest of us had missed.

Kitty Moore, senior editor at Guilford, suggested the need for several new chapters that immediately became the heart of the book.

Marie Sprayberry, copyeditor at Guilford, took a complicated manuscript and created a framework to support it.

Preface

In this book, I take one night in a life of a couple and, by detailing the half-thoughts and half-feelings that generally go unnoticed, I uncover everything I can about the couple's relationship—and, by extension, about all relationships.

The partners return home from work in the evening, and one of them says more about the problems of the day than the other wants to hear. Bit by bit, the evening unrolls. It is a composite drawn from what I have learned in my 26 years as a psychotherapist, my 18 years as a couples therapist, and—not least—my 25 years as a husband.

At several points in the evening, I stop the action and present a therapy session (either individual or couples) to demonstrate the therapeutic implications of what I am discussing. In addition to describing what happens in the therapy, I report the continuing conversation that I have with myself while doing therapy.

A skeptical reader pops up from time to time to challenge what I say. My relationship with this reader parallels that between the partners. Just as the partners struggle to work out some kind of reasonable relationship, so do the skeptic and I.

The discoveries I made while writing this book thus emerged out of four tensions: the momentum of the story, the momentum of the therapy sessions, my conversations with myself, and my debate with this skeptic.

Contents

CHAPTER 1

Major Points in the Book

Before describing this night in the life of a couple, I discuss the major principles of the book, some of which were present in my work before I started the writing and some of which have emerged, as you will see, during the writing.

- **None of us know what to do when something bothers us about our partners.** We can say something about it, but that just leads to bad feeling and fights. Or we can keep our mouths shut, but that just leads to a loss of feeling for our partners and, often to bad feeling and fights anyway when what we have suppressed eventually pops out. Those are our choices: We can say something and become alienated, or we can keep our mouths shut and become alienated.

This is the thesis with which I begin this book. I take a night in the life of a couple—Marie and Paul—and I describe their thoughts and feelings as they struggle with something that bothers each about the other. What quickly becomes clear is that their thoughts and feelings form an uninterrupted series of mental states with a life of their own.

- **Life is an uninterrupted series of states of mind over which we have little control.** Couple life is an uninterrupted series of couple states over which we as partners have little control. We do not choose our moods; we find ourselves in them. We do not choose our passions; our passions choose us.

I know that this differs from the current popular view, which is that people design their lives (at least unconsciously)—they make choices. This analysis of Marie and Paul's evening suggests that, instead, they pass through a continuing series of states of mind in which choice plays little part. For example:

At a certain moment in the evening, Marie snaps into the "It's-a-mistake-to-do-what-I'm-doing and-complain-that-Paul-doesn't-talk-enough, he's-just-going-to-feel-pressured, what-I'm-doing-is-only-making-things-worse" state of mind.

But once Marie establishes that what she is doing is counterproductive ("My pressuring Paul is only making things worse"), she immediately experiences it as a moral issue and herself as being on the low moral ground. She snaps into the "I-should-accept-people-the-way-they-are" state of mind.

And once she establishes that she should accept people the way they are, she immediately thinks that she is a person too and should accept herself the way *she* is. She snaps into the "I-have-a-right-to-my-wishes" state of mind.

And once she establishes that she has a right to her wishes, she immediately notices that her wishes aren't being fulfilled. She snaps into the "Paul-is-depriving-me" state of mind.

And once she establishes that Paul is depriving her, she immediately thinks that he must *want* to deprive her; she snaps into the "He's-enjoying-every-minute-of-this; he-wants-to-control-me" state of mind.

As this sequence suggests, an adequate description of a state of mind typically requires a string of phrases. As this sequence also suggests, a particular state of mind (e.g., "I have a right to my wishes") typically leads automatically to another (e.g., "And my wishes aren't being satisfied"). Snapping into another state of mind is like coming to the top of a mountain, whose vista opens upon the next mountain.

Marie does not choose the states of mind she passes through. She is only fleetingly aware of them and immediately forgets most of them. All she knows is that she suddenly feels abused and angry. And, feeling abused and angry, Marie temporarily loses her capacity to talk in a collaborative way.

• **People do not realize that their capacities come and go.** Our capacity to talk in a collaborative way and, for instance, to express feelings rather than make accusations—that is, to make "I statements" rather than "you statements"—requires being in the right state of mind. It is impossible to make "I statements" when you are in the "hating-my-partner, wanting-revenge, feeling-stung-and-needing-to-sting-back" state of mind. At such a moment, you cannot remember what an "I statement" is, and, frankly, you do not care.

We generally think of a capacity as something we have or do not have. Once we develop it, we have it forever, like riding a bike. But when it comes to capacities such as remaining objective, maintaining our sense of humor, empathizing with others, talking in a collaborative way, and making "I statements" rather than "you statements," we keep falling off the bike.

As you will read, at a certain point in one of Marie and Paul's therapy sessions with me, Marie snaps into the "feeling-angry, wanting-revenge" state of mind—which means that she loses her ability to make "I statements." She is unable to tell Paul, "Hmm, it's funny, but suddenly I'm enraged at you." Instead, she says, "You're selfish; you're irresponsible; you're trying to control me."

And, in response, Paul loses his ability to describe his experience—or even to know what it is. He is unable to say, "Wait a minute! We were just having this great talk and now suddenly you see me as the enemy. What happened?" Instead, he shrugs wearily and says nothing.

• **Our capacities *as therapists* come and go.** Being the kind of therapists we want to be requires being in a particular state of mind—and we cannot be in that state all the time.

Listening to Marie and Paul, I momentarily lose my capacities as a therapist. I snap into the "Marie-is-attacking-and-Paul-is-withdrawing, that-is-the-problem-they-came-in-with-and-I-haven't-been-able-to-help-them, I'm-not-doing-my-job, I'm-not-a-very-good-therapist" state of mind. By snapping into this state, I temporarily lose my ability to listen to them and to concentrate on what they say.

• **Whenever people are unable to get across their leading-edge feeling—and that is most of the time—they generate symptoms.** So they need a way to relate to themselves (and to their partners) as symptom-generating creatures.

As I show, symptoms emerge from our unavoidable failures to get across what we feel. I know that when we use the word "symptoms," we typically think of clearly maladaptive or pathological reactions such as insomnia, loss of appetite, and excessive drinking. But I am using the word in a broader way to include reactions such as flashes of sadness and lapses in concentration.

Here is the leading-edge feeling that Marie needs to get across:

> I really enjoyed the way we were talking, too—I felt closer to you than I have in a long time—but that just makes me aware of all the ways we're *not* close. And suddenly I feel furious—because at the moment I blame you for it.

Since Marie is unable to express this—or even to formulate it in her own mind—she has no choice but to experience it in vague, stuttering, and eruptive ways:

She suddenly feels sad without knowing why.
She has the momentary thought that maybe she should have married her previous boyfriend (even *with* his drinking problem).
She spews out, "You're selfish; you're irresponsible; you only think of yourself."

In other words, she generates symptoms, which sparks a leading-edge feeling in Paul that *he* now needs to get across. He needs to say:

Wait a minute! We were just having this great talk and now suddenly you're seeing me as the enemy. What happened?

Since he is unable to say this—or even to formulate it clearly to himself—Paul has no choice but to experience it in amorphous and fragmented ways:

He feels sorry that they have come for couples therapy tonight.
He wishes he were home watching *Monday Night Football.*
He really wants a cigarette (he gave up smoking a year ago).
He has a sudden desire to be up North fishing.
He shrugs wearily and says nothing.

In other words, Paul, too, has begun generating symptoms—which sparks a leading-edge feeling in me that *I* need to get across to myself. I need to be able to tell myself:

They're doing what they did when they first came to therapy. They've made no progress, I haven't helped them, I feel like an inadequate therapist—which means I'm in danger of temporarily losing my capacities as a therapist.

Since I am unable to say that to myself, I have no choice but to lose those capacities—that is, I too begin generating symptoms:

My mind wanders.
I have a sudden wish to be a carpenter so that I can see some progress after a day's work.
I feel weary.
For a moment, I think I may be coming down with the flu that is going around.

So there we are—the three of us—sitting in the office generating symptoms.

• As I have just shown, *not* getting across your leading-edge feeling leads to alienation. As I now show, getting across your leading-edge feeling leads to intimacy.

Intimacy is telling your partner the main thing on your mind and feeling that he or she understands, and it is your partner's telling you the same and feeling that *you* understand. It is getting across your leading-edge feeling to your partner and your partner's getting across his or her leading-edge feeling to you.

• In a fight, neither partner is able to make his or her point because it conflicts with the point that the other is trying to make—and that is what makes it a fight.

Marie wants Paul to agree that he should talk more about his feelings. But Paul will not agree. That is because it conflicts with his point, which is that it is better for him *not* to talk about his feelings, since when he does she just gets upset.

"You wouldn't talk about your feelings even if I didn't get upset," Marie tells him. "You're like your father—he never talks about anything—well, in his case nothing except bus schedules." Immediately the fight reorganizes around a new pair of points:

> Paul needs Marie to admit that he is not nearly as bad as his father before he will admit that he is somewhat like him.
> Marie needs Paul to admit that he is somewhat like his father before she will admit that Paul is not nearly as bad.

"I'm not like my father," Paul says. "I'm trying to change—and my father never did." With these words, the fight now reorganizes around yet another new pair of points:

> Paul needs Marie to acknowledge that he has been making an effort to change before he will admit that so far the change has not been great.
> Marie needs Paul to acknowledge that so far the change has not been great before she will admit that she knows he is trying to change.

Whatever new point one partner tries to make immediately draws a conflicting point from the other.

• Part of fighting is insisting that *you* are not fighting but that your partner is.

Marie says, "You're being defensive." Paul says, "No I'm not; you're being critical." Marie says, "I'm not being critical; I'm just telling you how I feel."

Suddenly Marie and Paul are no longer fighting about any of the issues but, instead, about who is responsible for the fight and about who is behaving more unreasonably. In fact, *that* is the new issue.

Paul would be shocked if Marie were to become nondefensive and, for example, were to answer his charge, "You're being critical," with this: "Hmm. I guess I am. And that's too bad, because there was something important I wanted to tell you." Marie would be shocked if Paul were to answer her charge, "You're being defensive," in a nondefensive and nonattacking manner by saying, "You could be right about that. And I could see how that wouldn't help matters." In both cases, Marie and Paul would be stepping back from the precipice and onto a "platform" from which to view the situation.

- **Mental life to a large extent is a struggle for self-justification.**

In looking at the fine texture of Marie and Paul's evening—their moods, exchanges, disputes, and symptoms—we discover that a key element is self-blame.

Marie tells herself, "I'm selfish, demanding, and needy; I shouldn't be trying to force Paul to talk more." Then, engaging in self-justification, she tells herself:

I have a right to my feelings too.
The problem isn't my neediness—it's Paul's failure to give me what I deserve.
I can't be all bad. I have two wonderful children and a career, and I'm really good at making friends.
Anyway, I'm less demanding than I used to be.

Paul blames himself too. He tells himself, "I don't talk to Marie as much as I should. I let her down. I don't give her what she deserves. There's something wrong with me—I'm too detached." Then, engaging in self-justification, he adds:

I work hard all day; I need time to unwind.
The problem isn't my failure to give Marie what she deserves—it's her neediness.
I can't be all bad. I bring in a good paycheck.
And, anyway, I talk more than I used to.

The mind is "a self-justifying organ," observed Bernard Apfelbaum, my authority on ego analysis—the theoretical orientation underlying this book.

• **The source of all the problems described above (and the supraordinate idea in this book) is feeling unentitled to feelings.**

On any given day, people have certain feelings that they feel ashamed of—that is, that they judge themselves to be weak, bad, crazy, immature, unmanly, or unfeminine for having. They react to such judgment by behaving in all the ways I just described. They do the following:

1. Lose the ability to get these feelings across.
2. Generate symptoms.
3. Snap into alienated states of mind.
4. Experience a decreased sense of intimacy.
5. Lose their capacities and, in particular, their ability to think.
6. Become self-blaming.

In response to their self-blaming, people do two further things:

7. Engage in self-justification.
8. Blame their partners, which, if expressed, typically leads to fighting or withdrawal.

Fighting is frustrating because:

9. Neither partner is able to make his or her point.
10. Everything becomes part of the fight, including the fighting itself; that is, part of fighting is insisting that *you* are not fighting but that your partner is.

To avoid fighting (because it *is* so frustrating and because it leads to so many problems), partners:

11. Try to keep their mouths shut. But that just leads to withdrawal, and, eventually, to blurting things out anyway. In other words, "We can criticize our partners and become alienated, or we can keep our mouths shut and become alienated; those are our choices."

• **An appreciation of all these factors—and how they emerge from a feeling of unentitlement—leads to a therapeutic approach based on the following four principles:**

The "platform" principle. The goal of therapy is to establish a platform—a nonaccusing vantage point—from which clients can monitor all the things I have just described: how they feel unentitled to their feelings, shift among states of mind, lose their capacities, lose their ability to think, generate symptoms, struggle for self-justification, and so on.

The "need-to-get-something-across" principle. The task at any given moment in a therapy session is to discover what the client needs to get across in order to stop generating symptoms.

The "hidden-validity" principle. Another task is to discover the invalidating (self-discrediting, self-reproaching) idea that leads to the client's feeling unentitled to his or her feelings and resulting inability to get them across.

The "victim" principle. The master and capping self-invalidating idea is "I'm doing it to myself." In telling themselves this, clients are blaming themselves for their problems. Instead of appreciating how they are victims—that is, how they are trapped, stuck, and deprived—they accuse themselves of unconsciously wanting the problems that beset them, of even "creating" them, and of getting too much from their symptoms to be willing to give them up.

• **Here is how these four therapeutic principles follow from the supraordinate "sense-of-entitlement" idea.** As a result of feeling *un*entitled to their feelings, clients do the following:

Discount, disqualify, dismiss, discredit, impugn, or otherwise invalidate their feelings—which I deal with therapeutically by focusing on what is valid in their reactions (the "hidden-validity" principle).

Are unable to get their feelings across—which I deal with therapeutically by trying to figure out at any given moment what they need to get across to stop generating symptoms (the "need-to-get-something-across" principle).

Conclude that their problems are their own fault ("I'm doing it to myself")—which I deal with therapeutically by recognizing how they are stuck, trapped, and deprived; that is, how they are victims (the "victim" principle).

Are unable to establish a platform (a neutral, objective, non-blame-oriented, nondefensive, nonanxious vantage point) from which to monitor their feelings and problems—which I deal with therapeutically by providing glimpses of such a platform (the "platform" principle).

These four principles, along with the supraordinate "sense-of-entitlement-to-feelings" idea, constitute the theory of thinking and the approach to therapy upon which this book is based: ego analysis. Having an ego-analytic approach *means* viewing clients with these four principles and this idea in mind. In this book, I focus on two of these principles: the "platform" and "need-to-get-something-across" principles. The other two—the "hidden validity" and "victim" principles—are implied. All four are discussed in Chapter 27.

My goal in this book is to present an extended, detailed, clinically useful example of ego-analytic thinking. This model of the mind has its roots in Freud (1926/1959), emerged in the work of Otto Fenichel (1941), and was further developed by Paul Gray (1982) and Bernard Apfelbaum (Apfelbaum, 1977, 1982b, 1988; Apfelbaum & Apfelbaum, 1985; Apfelbaum & Gill, 1989). My own work (Wile, 1981, 1984, 1985a, 1985b, 1987, 1988, in press-a, in press-b) follows the line of thinking developed by Apfelbaum.

Ego analysis is not to be confused with Hartmann's and Rapaport's ego psychology. As Apfelbaum (1966, 1983) has demonstrated, ego psychology is an extension of id-analytic thinking, whereas ego analysis is an alternative to it.

Here is ego-analytic thinking in a nutshell: In addition to the obvious problem that the client comes in and tells you about, there is always a hidden problem, which is the client's intolerance of the obvious problem—in particular, the client's "anxious, discouraged, despairing, counterphobic, self-accusing, unable-to-tolerate-having-the-problem, anxiously-trying-to-solve-it-or-to-brush-it-away, flinching" reaction to the obvious problem. Taken together, such responses constitute an inability to "have" the problem, or, to say the same thing in another way, to feel "entitled" to it.

Ego analysis is about this ability or inability to "have" a problem—or a feeling or experience:

> We feel sad and we think we should not feel sad (we feel unentitled to our sadness). We tell ourselves: "Being sad doesn't help. I shouldn't let things get to me the way I do. I should be able to look on the positive side. And, anyway, I should be over it by now."
> We feel angry, and we think we should not feel angry (we feel unentitled to our anger) because we feel we have insufficient justification for it; thus, we suppress it. But then, some time later, we blurt it out in a more eruptive and provocative form than if we had expressed the anger directly in the first place. Feeling unentitled to a feeling (in this case, anger) has produced a problem. But we also feel unentitled to the problem—that is, we see ourselves as "weak," "inhibited," or "immature" for having the problem of suppressing our anger and then blurting it out. We fail to recognize that suppression, which then leads to blurting,

is unavoidable. Everyone is repeatedly going to suppress. Suppression is unavoidable because "feeling unentitled to feelings," the major *cause* of suppression, is itself ultimately unavoidable.

As these examples suggest, life is to an important extent the relationship we have with ourselves about our feelings, experiences, and problems—following, in large part, from our ability or inability to have, inhabit, or feel entitled to them. As these examples also suggest, the major contributor to the feeling of *un*entitlement is self-reproach (i.e., shame, guilt, superego injunctions, negative self-talk, self-blame, self-criticism, and self-hate). Self-reproach shuts down productive thinking; it impairs a person's problem-solving ability, much as an immune deficiency impairs the ability to fight disease.

A therapist who adopts such a stance is alert to ways in which his or her interventions may feed into a client's self-reproach. The therapist's task is to help create a platform from which clients can monitor the problem of their inability to "have," "inhabit," or feel "entitled" to their feelings, experiences, and problems.

Before beginning my description of Marie and Paul's evening, I introduce the skeptical reader who, as I have said in the Preface, pops up from time to time to object to what I say.

Skeptic: And I have an objection already—to your remark about "keeping your mouth shut and becoming alienated." I don't think that keeping your mouth shut is always such a bad idea.

Wile: I don't either.

Skeptic: But didn't you say that keeping your mouth shut leads to trouble, since it produces withdrawal and eventually you're going to blurt things out anyway?

Wile: Well, yes, but *not* keeping your mouth shut can lead to more immediate and more certain trouble.

Skeptic: But don't you believe in communication? I thought all therapists believed in communication.

Wile: If people don't have a *way* to talk, communicating just leads to problems.

Skeptic: Yes, that's what I say—we should keep our mouths shut.

Wile: But of course, keeping our mouths shut *also* leads to problems.

Skeptic: But it doesn't have to. I don't say anything to my friend Sally about her chewing with her mouth open, or to my friend Ben about his habit of interrupting. I ignore those things—they *don't* create problems. I let them roll off my back. And I *don't* eventually blurt them out.

Wile: That's what's good about friends. They're not as important to you as someone you live with and spend a lot of time with. So you can often ignore their faults. But suppose Sally were your roommate. Or suppose you went on a long trip with her. The way she chews might eventually get to you—and you *might* blurt something out. And suppose Ben were your *husband* . . .

Skeptic: Well, actually, my husband is *like* Ben—he interrupts me. It drives me crazy sometimes. And—well, yes, okay—maybe I *do* blurt things out.

Wile: I'm not surprised. It's hard to let things roll off your back when it's your *partner*.

Skeptic: But my husband's a special case—you never saw anyone so stubborn.

Wile: Everyone's husband is a "special case." And so is everyone's wife. After spending the entire day showing partners how to reason with each other, I come home to find the one person in the world you *can't* reason with: my wife, Joanne. She's a special case. And Joanne, who's a therapist herself and also spends the day working with people, thinks that *I'm* a special case—that there's no reasoning with me.

Skeptic: But you never met my husband—he *is* a special case.

Wile: Let me tell you about Marie and Paul, then—because each of them thinks the other is a special case.

BLAMING YOURSELF

Marie and Paul, the main characters in this book, are in their early 30s, have been married for ten years, and have two children, Billy, 7, and Jeannie, 3.[1] It is early evening. Paul has just come home from work. Marie, who came home earlier, greets him at the door.

Most of the action in Part 1 takes place in Marie's head (later I describe what goes on in Paul's):

In Chapter 2, we notice *how much* goes on in her head.

In Chapter 3, we discover that she needs to talk to Paul to more fully figure out what goes on in her head.

In Chapter 4, we notice that much of what goes on in her head is self-blame.

In Chapter 5, we notice that much of Marie's life—and, by extension, everyone's life—is devoted to *self-justification* to deal with self-blame.

Throughout Part 1, we observe that Marie continually shifts among states of mind. This fact leads in Part 2 to a therapeutic approach devoted to creating a nonaccusing vantage point—a platform—from which Marie can monitor these shifts.

---

[1]Marie and Paul are heterosexual, are married, and have children. But I could as easily have used as my example partners who are gay or lesbian, are unmarried, or have no children. The principles would be the same.

CHAPTER 2

The Ongoing Conversation
We Have with Ourselves

There is a lot more going on in everyone's head than anyone realizes.

Paul has just come home, and Marie has a lot to tell him:

> You won't believe what my boss did today. She gave me the
> *Rodriguez* file—that's *her* account. My boss makes twice my salary,
> does half the work, and now she's palming off even that. And then
> she has the nerve to complain about my not immediately getting
> to it—as if that's the only work I had to do today. I couldn't wait
> to get home—though things weren't much better here. Brenda [the
> sitter] said the kids were fighting all afternoon. And when I went
> into the kitchen to start dinner, your darling daughter Jeannie,
> who was *supposed* to be taking her nap, got into the photos from
> our trip and started to paste them together. And when I discov-
> ered what she was doing and began scraping off the paste, Billy
> wandered into the hall and, as you can see, started a mural on
> the walls.

Marie is *about* to go on to tell Paul that when she went downstairs
to find something to clean crayon off walls, she found the basement
swarming with insects—she is afraid they are termites. But she notices
a slight twitch in Paul's upper lip, which she has learned is a sign that
he does not want to hear any more.

Marie is doing something remarkable here. Take a thousand people
off the street and put them in her place—none of them would know what
the twitch in Paul's upper lip means. They would not even notice the
twitch. Marie is the world's leading expert on Paul's nonverbal behav-

ior. His mother, his sister, and his best friend, Mark, are good at it. But
Marie is the best. Scientists cannot teach computers to do what Marie
has just done.

Of course, at the moment Marie is not thinking of herself as an
expert. She just feels hurt. She wants to talk to Paul, but Paul does not
want to talk to her. So she sorts through the following possibilities:

> I'll talk in a more entertaining way. But no, whenever I try to do
> that, it comes out awkward.
>
> I'll tell Paul I'm hurt that he doesn't want to listen. But no, he'll
> deny it. He'll say he *does* want to listen, and I'll just feel frustrated.
>
> I'll give him time to relax and try to talk to him later. No, there
> isn't going to be a later. By the time we get the kids to bed and
> clean up, we'll both be too tired.
>
> I'll finish what I want to say *now*, but I'll do it *fast*, so it won't bother
> him so much. No, I won't—that's begging for scraps of attention.
>
> I'll ask how *his* day went—and hope that will put him in a mood to
> listen to the rest of mine. That's not a great plan. He'll probably
> just say "Pretty good," and sit down and watch the News. But I
> can't think of anything better.

Now, you might think it would take a long time for Marie to sort
through all these possibilities. But she does it standing in the hall in
less time than it would take to scratch an itch. And after all this thinking, here is what she says:

> Well, how did things go for *you* today?

We are all closet Einsteins. The mundane things we say make it easy
to miss the high-powered thinking that goes into them. Marie does not
feel very much like an Einstein, however, since in answer to her "How
did things go for *you* today?", Paul says:

> Pretty good; I'm just a little tired.

And he goes into the living room to watch the News—which is
exactly what she was afraid of. Marie feels rejected. Her desire to tell
him about her day is immediately replaced by a more modest wish—to
hear something friendly from him to relieve this feeling of rejection.
She suppresses the urge to chase after him, though—that does not seem
dignified. And, anyway, it never works—it just leads to his digging himself in further. So she stands there not knowing what to do.

Marie's conversation with Paul has ended, but not the ongoing one she is having with herself, which is by far more interesting anyway—although, as is true of most of our inner dialogues, it goes by too fast for it to register fully.

The Tangle of Voices in Marie's Head

What's wrong with me that Paul doesn't want to talk to me?

What's wrong with *Paul* that he can't listen to three words from his wife without immediately turning on the TV?

The man's tired. Give him a break. Customers have been after him all day.

I'll give him a break. I'll break his leg. I hate it when he runs from me. I told him I had an awful day. He should have been more understanding. At the very least, he should have offered to make dinner.

But he made dinner the *last three nights.*

So, it would *hurt* him to make it a *fourth*?

Well, he *might* have if I hadn't *jumped* him. He'd hardly taken his coat off before I started telling him about my boss, the kids, and everything else.

They're his kids too—he ought to be interested.

He *is* interested. I've just got to stop being so dependent and running to him for every little thing.

Why is it so dependent to want a little conversation with your husband?

I expect him to drop whatever he wants to do and listen to me. That's selfish.

I'll tell you what's selfish: refusing to listen to your wife when she's had a bad day. He doesn't care about me. He doesn't care about the family. All he cares about is the store. He's married to that store. He doesn't know how to have a relationship—he's afraid of commitment, and he's still hung up on his mother.

Maybe he just has different needs than you do. You can't expect him to be exactly like you.

That's just the problem—we're so *very* different. We probably should never have gotten married.

If you married someone else there would still be problems. They'd just be *different* ones. You have to learn to accept Paul the way he is.

But suppose I *can't* accept him the way he is?

What an evolutionary achievement to produce a creature who can think like this! Of course, Marie is not viewing her thinking as an evolutionary achievement. She just feels bad. In the course of these thoughts, Marie shifts back and forth between blaming herself, which leaves her feeling depressed, and blaming Paul, which leaves her feeling lonely and scared. And when she *stops* blaming and considers the possibility that she and Paul simply have different needs, she ends up with the panicky thought that the two of them are incompatible and should never have married. And when she tries to relieve the growing panic by reminding herself that there are *always* problems in a relationship, she ends up lecturing herself about her need to accept Paul the way he is, which discourages her, because at the moment she is not sure she *can* accept him.

Skeptic: Marie sounds pretty neurotic.
Wile: That's what Marie would think too—if she were aware of all her thoughts. But she's *un*aware of most of them. They go by too fast. She catches only a half-thought here and there, and then quickly forgets most of those. This is how everyone's mind works. We all have such inner dialogues of which we are only partly aware.

This description of Marie's inner dialogue is a CAT scan into the mind. It reveals the kinds of thoughts and feelings that everyone always has but that typically remain invisible. There is a lot more going on in everyone's head than anyone ever realizes.

CHAPTER 3

Using Our Relationship
to Figure Out What We Feel

Feeling that someone is on your side can help you get on your own side.

Marie wants to talk to Paul, but he has disappeared to watch the News. And she has another problem: She does not know exactly what she wants to talk about. She *thinks* she knows. She thinks she wants to tell him about her difficult boss, the crayoned walls, the sticky pictures, the termites, and so on. And she *does* want to tell him about these things. But she wants to tell him something even more important. The problem is, the only way she can figure out what it is is *by* talking to him.

So let us have her talk to him. Let us imagine what would happen if Paul's lip were *not* to twitch and if, after listening to what she has to say, he were to tell her:

Poor Marie, you've had a hard day.

Let us imagine further what would happen if Marie were to take his comment, not as condescending, but as sympathizing—that is, as showing that he is on her side. After her difficult day, it would be a comfort to feel that someone is on her side. She might fight back tears.

Feeling that Paul is on her side would enable Marie to get more on her own side—that is, to feel sufficiently entitled to her feelings to begin to figure out what they are. She would say:

You know, it's not just today. Things have gotten completely out of hand. I've been feeling overwhelmed for a while now.

Marie would not have *known* that she has been feeling overwhelmed lately. Having heard what she said, now she would. Telling Paul about

19

the crayoned walls, the termites, and so on (and feeling he understands) would allow her to discover that she has been feeling generally over-whelmed lately. And saying this (and feeling that Paul understands) would allow her to go on to the next discovery:

MARIE: You know, what bothers me most is that we hardly have any time for each other. We both know that I wouldn't trade Jeannie and Billy for anything, but having them means that we have no money, no time, and no relationship. I'm beginning to wonder who that strange man is who gets into bed with me every night.
PAUL: I think he's me. But I've been feeling so overwhelmed myself lately that I'm not completely sure.

Here is the point: Relationships offer opportunities to express the feelings that have been generated within us during the day, but they also offer opportunities to discover what these feelings are. Paul's sym-pathetic "Poor Marie, you've really had a hard day," would enable her to sympathize sufficiently with herself to discover that she has been feeling overwhelmed and disconnected from him.

Paul would be touched that Marie is touched by what he has just said. Marie's warm response to his comment would enable him to feel warm and sympathetic enough toward himself to be able to figure out more of what *he* feels. He would say:

This isn't the way it was supposed to be. I thought having kids would bring us closer, not make us strangers. How did this happen to us?

And now the tears might stream down Marie's face, and Paul might be on the verge of crying too. They would experience the intimacy that can come from confiding in each other about their lack of intimacy.

This sounds like a different Paul from the one in Chapter 2. It is the man the Paul from Chapter 2 would *like* to be. It is the Paul that we would *all* like to be. Everyone would enjoy being able to reach through to his or her partner in this way.

Skeptic: But don't you think there's something wrong with Marie for having to rely on Paul to figure out what she feels? I'm beginning to think that maybe she *is* too dependent on him, just as she says.
Wile: I don't think you appreciate how hard it can be to figure out what you feel.
Skeptic: I don't see how it's so hard to figure out that you feel over-

whelmed by your life and disconnected from your husband. I've already done it three times this week.

    Wile: Well, you must have been in a particularly "able-to-take-my-own-side, feeling-sympathetic-toward-myself" state of mind, since, as I'm saying, that is what it typically takes.

    Marie is not in a "self-sympathetic" state of mind, however. Remember, she is trying to fight off self-blame. She says to herself:

> Jeannie's starting to be uncontrollable: pasting together our photos from the trip.
> She's just inquisitive. All kids are like that. She's just going through a stage.
> I'm tired of that stage.
> You're tired of *every* stage. What's your problem? Mothers have been bringing up children for millions of years without half the complaining you do in an hour. As for Jeannie getting into the photos, it's your own fault; for one thing, you should have watched her more carefully, and for another, you should have put the photos in a safer place.
> You can't watch a 3-year-old every minute, and you can't lock up everything you own.
> Maybe not, but you should have known that something was up when things suddenly got so quiet.
> I thought Jeannie was taking a nap, and Billy was coloring. I had no idea that he was collecting his crayons for an assault on the hall.
> That's another thing. Don't you think you overreacted just a little—telling Billy he can't go to the ballgame with his dad?
> Ile's got to be taught a lesson.
> Telling him he can't go to the ballgame isn't going to teach him a lesson; it's going to teach him to hate his mother.

    In this inner debate, Marie is unable to adopt the "self-sympathetic, taking-my-own-side" attitude she needs in order to discover that she has been feeling overwhelmed and disconnected from Paul lately.

    Skeptic: But Marie *is* taking her own side. She's saying, "You can't watch a 3-year-old every minute." She's saying, "He's got to be taught a lesson." I call that taking her own side.

    Wile: But when she tells herself, "You can't watch a 3-year-old every minute," she's defending herself against the self-blaming thought, "You *should* have watched her more carefully." And when she tells herself, "He's got to be taught a lesson," she's defending herself against the self-blaming thought, "Maybe my punishment was too harsh." What looks like "taking her own side" is really defending against self-attack. There is a war going on in her head in which she is trying to fight off self-blame by justifying her behavior. In other words, what on the surface looks like "taking her own side" is the result of her *failure* to take her own side. It is the result of her inability to adopt a "self-sympathetic, giving-myself-the-benefit-of-the-doubt" attitude in the first place.

It is hard for Marie to sympathize with herself when she is worried about being a bad mother. Given her "self-accusing" state of mind, she would never think to say to herself, "Poor Marie, you've had a hard day." She needs somebody else to say it for her. And it would shock her to hear Paul say it, since it is so foreign to the way she is thinking.

But it would be *wonderful* to hear.

And Paul would be able to say it because he would have a more sympathetic view of Marie than her view of herself—Paul would *not* be seeing her as a bad mother. Marie could then piggyback on Paul's more positive attitude toward her.

A major value of relationships is that they can at times provide a more self-accepting atmosphere than people can provide for themselves, and, by doing so, can free their thinking. In this new, more self-accepting atmosphere, Marie would be able to realize that she feels *angry* at the kids. She would allow herself to express to Paul the daringly unmotherly thought:

> I know I said I wouldn't trade our kids for anything, but I wonder what we could get for them.

A moment ago, Marie was operating under this principle: "You should never resent your kids no matter what." This interchange with Paul would allow her to shift to a more self-tolerant principle: "It is normal at times to resent your kids."

PAUL: I wouldn't count on getting very much for them. The market isn't very good these days for household vandals under the age of 7. We'd have to *pay* to get them off our hands.

MARIE (*laughing*): How much?

Suddenly Marie would feel better. Having said how much she resents her kids, she would find herself no longer resenting them. In fact, Jeannie and Billy would begin to seem lovable again. Jeannie, who a moment ago seemed an evil child committed to the destruction of everything of value in the house, would begin to seem inventive and imaginative. And Billy, who a moment ago was the graffiti artist from hell, would now seem like an indefatigable creative spirit. They would not have changed; Marie's feelings about them would have changed. Being a good mother appears to include an ability not to feel too bad for having the wish at times to trade in your kids.

CHAPTER 4

Self-Blame

The internal debate in which Marie engages—and in which all of us engage—suggests, not so much the zip-zip of the supercomputer, as I earlier suggested, as the clank-clank of an badly out of tune engine. The mind is efficient in some ways and inefficient in others. As I shall show in this chapter, the inefficiency emerges, in large part, from our ongoing battle with our harsh internal critic.

The Paul that Marie would *like*—and *any* partner would like—is a Paul who listens to her and helps her figure out what she feels. But the Paul she has is plopped down watching the News and, as far as she can tell, hoping to hear no more from her for the rest of the evening, at the minimum.

So what does she do? She goes into the kitchen to fix dinner.

But Paul's withdrawal has dispirited her. Her ongoing conversation with herself—which had already taken a sour turn (from discussion to debate)—now takes another (from debate to self-persecution):

Marie's Self-Persecution

You should be stripped of your mother's stripes—getting upset because the kids were fighting. That's what kids do—fight. You've heard of sibling rivalry, haven't you?

So they messed up the walls and the photos a little. What do you want them to do at their age—sit quietly and plan for the future?

You shouldn't take out on them the anger you're really feeling toward your boss.

And you shouldn't be so angry at her. You shouldn't let her get to you like that.

And it was crazy to try to comfort yourself with a chocolate donut. You're supposed to be on a diet.

And you *certainly* shouldn't have had a *second*. Haven't you got even a modicum of self-control?

You have no judgment either or you wouldn't have tried to make up for it by taking that extra exercise class at lunchtime. It's your own fault your back started hurting again.

And if that weren't stupid enough, you had to blurt out every gory detail to Paul before he even had a chance to take his coat off. It's your own fault he disappeared into the living room.

Skeptic: I told you Marie's neurotic. Why is she being so hard on herself? She's the most conscience-stricken person I've ever seen.

Wile: She's slipped into the kind of awful mood in which you can't think of anything that isn't a self-criticism.

Skeptic: I don't get into such moods.

Wile: You're the first person in history, then, because everyone does—although some people don't know when they're in them. They just feel gloomy or distracted and can't figure out why. They're unaware of the underlying thoughts. Marie *is* aware of those thoughts. And what her thoughts reveal is that she—and, by inference, all of us—come equipped with harsh taskmasters rapping our knuckles with rulers. Each rap is a moral injunction:

You shouldn't have been so harsh with the kids. (*Rap.*)
You're a bad mother. (*Rap.*)
You shouldn't take out on them your anger at your boss. (*Rap.*)
You shouldn't let your boss get to you. (*Rap.*)
You shouldn't have gone off your diet. (*Rap.*)
You've no self-control. You're weak. (*Rap.*)
You're too dependent. (*Rap.*)
You're a nag. (*Rap.*)
Bottom line: You've only yourself to blame. (*Rap-Rap.*)

What is worse is that Marie does not think of these statements as moral injunctions. She thinks of them as truths. We are so used to standing in judgment of our feelings and reactions that we are unaware of doing so. We are convinced that we are just describing reality.

As I see it, everyone's root problem is the presence of these moral injunctions—this self-reproach, self-blame, self-hate, shame, guilt, negative self-talk (spoken in this harsh internal voice)—and, more generally, feeling unentitled to certain feelings.

Skeptic: Aren't you being a little simplistic here? Plenty of people—like me, for instance—are hardly ever self-blaming. So how can you say that self-reproach is *everyone's* root problem?

Wile: Because self-reproach typically reveals itself, not directly, but by its *effects*. People become demoralized, distracted, or withdrawn; they lose the ability to think objectively; they—

Skeptic: I don't do any of those things.

Wile: Well, *another* way that self-reproach reveals itself is through the effort to *relieve* it—people engage in defensive or self-justification efforts; they blame others to get the blame off themselves; they—

Skeptic: Well, okay, maybe, once in a blue moon, I do blame somebody who doesn't deserve it. But you still haven't proven that self-reproach is everyone's root problem. And you haven't said anything about how you think we *get* this way.

Wile: We *start* this way. Children instinctively blame themselves. They think it's their fault if their father dies or if their parents get a divorce. They feel it's because they've been bad.

Skeptic: But that's what we do when we're *children*. As adults we don't think that way.

Wile: Even for us as adults, self-reproach has an insistent, oppressive, all-encompassing quality. As soon as someone suggests to us that we are dependent, selfish, defensive, or, lately, *co*dependent, we immediately feel the weight of public opinion against us. We feel the weight of our *own* opinion against us.

Skeptic: Yes, but—

Wile: And being accused is being convicted. Once you are labeled defensive, codependent, and so on, you find it hard to defend yourself. Everyone just immediately thinks it is true about you.

Mental life is, to a large extent, seeking ways to deal with self-reproach—these harsh internal taskmasters that we might not even know we have. One way is by using our partners as confidants. If Paul were to say, "Poor Marie, you've really had a hard day," Marie's harsh taskmaster might immediately disappear—Marie might begin to see herself in a forgiving rather than in a self-accusing way.

How can such a powerful malevolent force as the harsh internal taskmaster so quickly disappear? Because relationships provide an equally powerful *curative* force.

But what happens if we do not have a partner or friend to talk to? And what happens if our partner or friend doesn't protect us from our internal taskmaster's moral injunctions but instead *reinforces* them—or worse, contributes *new* ones that our internal taskmaster hadn't yet thought of?

At the moment Marie is in such a situation—no one is around to protect her from her harsh internal taskmaster:

Paul is unavailable—he is watching the News.

Marie's friend Nancy is also unavailable—she is on the way home from work.

Marie's sister Sarah *is* available. But if Marie were to call her, Sarah would say, "You're becoming more like Mom all the time—yelling at your kids and nagging Paul." In so saying, Sarah would be joining forces with Marie's taskmaster.

Marie is in a life-long battle with her taskmaster—as all of us are with ours. Marie might be able to decrease this taskmaster's influence on her, but she will not be able to eliminate it entirely.

CHAPTER 5

Self-Justification: Fighting Off Self-Blame

Mental life is, to an important extent, an ongoing effort at self-justification to deal with self-blame.

What do people do when, like Marie, they are harangued by their harsh internal voice and there is no one there to help? They run for cover. They take a warm bath, go to bed and pull the covers over them, go to a movie, watch television, go shopping, run around the block, clean out their closets, change the oil in the car—anything to distract themselves and drown out their internal taskmaster's voice.

Of course, Marie does not have time to do any of these things—she is making dinner. So she does the only thing she can think of to distract herself; she switches on the radio.

And that turns out to be a good move. An author is being interviewed about her new book, *Supermom*, which describes women who try to do it all: be a perfect wife and mother, hold down a job, and organize the household. Hearing the difficulties these other women have—they do not appear to handle the pressures any better than she does—Marie begins to sympathize with herself for all she has to deal with.

Marie's harsh internal taskmaster continues to make charges. Emboldened by her increased sympathy for herself, however, Marie is better able to defend herself:

THE TASKMASTER'S CHARGE: You shouldn't have been so hard on Billy and Jeannie today.

MARIE'S DEFENSE: They have to be taught to respect other people's property.

THE TASKMASTER'S CHARGE: A mother should be understanding; children need love, and eventually they'll grow out of it.
MARIE'S DEFENSE: Children need limits, or they'll never grow out of it.

And now we can see what this shift in Marie's state of mind can do: It can make available ideas that a moment before were unavailable. Marie now has "truths" to dispute her internal taskmaster's "truths."

THE TASKMASTER'S CHARGE: Your kids are just going to learn to hate their mother.
MARIE'S DEFENSE: The purpose of being a mother isn't to win popularity contests.

THE TASKMASTER'S CHARGE: There's another reason you shouldn't express your anger. When you yell at your kids, you're teaching them that yelling is okay, and when they're parents, they're just going to yell at their *own* kids.
MARIE'S DEFENSE: What's wrong with that? Kids need to be taught that anger is part of life so that they won't be afraid of it.

THE TASKMASTER'S CHARGE: It doesn't *have* to be a part of life. For one thing, you shouldn't be so affected by what your boss does.
MARIE'S DEFENSE: You shouldn't *put up* with what your boss does. You should assert your rights.

THE TASKMASTER'S CHARGE: Okay, you *shouldn't* put up with what your boss does—you're chicken.
MARIE'S DEFENSE: Why do something stupid and impulsive and get yourself fired?

THE TASKMASTER'S CHARGE: Speaking of stupid and impulsive—you're a pig, scarfing down those donuts.
MARIE'S DEFENSE: Life is too short to spend forever dieting.

THE TASKMASTER'S CHARGE: You're too dependent. Not just on donuts either. You lean on Paul too much.
MARIE'S DEFENSE: No one is an island. A person shouldn't be afraid to ask for a little help when she needs it.

THE TASKMASTER'S CHARGE: What about *Paul's* needs? You're only thinking about yours. You're selfish.
MARIE'S DEFENSE: It's *important* to think about your needs and not sacrifice them to everyone else's.

Marie's internal taskmaster is using conventional wisdom—sayings that everyone in our culture accepts as true—as a weapon against her.

He is putting her down in ways that are difficult to defend against. How can Marie answer the charges that she is selfish, dependent, a pig?

How? By using cultural sayings of her own in her defense. Life is, to an important extent, a fighting off of moral injunctions by appealing to other moral injunctions. That is what much of our "thinking" is.

Appealing to moral injunctions to fight off moral injunctions is a way of relating to yourself that I call "justifying." Marie is "justifying" when she tells herself:

> I didn't yell at the kids that much, and anyway, it's for their own good: They've got to learn that they can't always do exactly what they want just because they feel like it.

Why do I call this "justifying" when it just seems the normal kind of reasoning that everyone uses without even thinking about it—and, furthermore, when the statement seems at least partly true? After all, kids *do* have to learn that they cannot always do as they please.

I call it "justifying" because Marie is fighting something off. She is not thinking about the issue in an unbiased and objective way. She is trying to convince herself of something; she is defending herself against the charge that she yelled at her kids too much.

Here is what Marie might say to herself if she were *not* justifying—that is, if she were not blaming herself and, as a result, had no need to defend herself:

> Poor me—what bad luck to have my resources low on a day that the kids decide to get creative. And what a shame that I have to end up feeling like a bad mother.

Instead of saying, "No, no; I didn't do it; I didn't yell at the kids and, anyway, they had it coming"—that is, instead of defending herself—Marie would be sympathizing with herself.

Skeptic: I don't think she *should* be sympathizing with herself. All that "poor me" and "what a shame" stuff is self-indulgent. Marie should take responsibility for what she does rather than making excuses and blaming it all on the kids.

Wile: But she *wouldn't* be blaming it all on the kids—as we can see by what she would tell herself next:

> And poor Billy and Jeannie—just their luck to catch me on a day when I've been preoccupied with problems at work. Of course, maybe they've been acting up *because* I've been preoccupied and

haven't paid much attention to them. In that case, poor *us*—the kids get neglected and yelled at, and I feel bad for neglecting and yelling.

It is a rare and special state of mind in which a mother is able to sympathize with herself for having to deal with her kids, and, at the same time, to sympathize with them for having to deal with her. It is generally not thought possible to do both.

It is a rare and special state of mind, and, unfortunately, Marie is not in it. As I have said, she is in a "justifying" state of mind—she is trying to fight off self-blame. And she doesn't succeed, which leaves her with an empty feeling and an urge to eat something more. So she finishes off the potato chips that the kids had for their snack—which immediately thrusts her back into the "self-hating" state of mind:

> The pig strikes again; two donuts this morning and now these chips. (*Rap.*)

Which she deals with by shifting back into the "justifying" state of mind:

> Why should I have to starve myself just because the fashion magazines want women to look anorexic?

This is not a bad defense, if Marie can hold onto it. Unfortunately, because of the influence of her harsh internal taskmaster, she cannot. She quickly falls back into the "self-hating" state of mind:

> I'll be a blimp in a week if I keep this up.

So here is the situation we are all in: We try to justify our reactions in an effort to snap out of the "non-self-sympathetic, self-hating" state of mind. What we would really like, of course, is not to have to justify anything, but to be in the "self-sympathetic" state of mind automatically. If Marie were in such a state of mind, here is what she might tell herself:

> It's a good thing chocolate donuts and potato chips were invented, because after what happened with my boss this morning, the kids this evening, and Paul just now, I really need something to cheer me up.

(If Marie were able to say this to herself, of course, she would have more pleasure eating these chips.)

Now I know it is *hard* to imagine Marie (or anyone) being able to talk to herself in this way, given cultural views about eating, dieting, and self-control. So let us try the next best thing and imagine Marie sympathizing with herself for being *unable* to sympathize with herself:

> What a shame that, in addition to going off my diet—which is disappointing because I'd been so pleased with myself for staying on it—I'm beating myself up for it.

Now, I know it is hard to imagine Marie (or anyone) being able to talk to herself in this way either, since it involves beating herself up and, at the same time, sympathizing with herself for beating herself up. But that is my goal: to create a "non-self-blaming" vantage point from which Marie can view these inevitable periods of self-blame.

We continually shift into and out of different states of mind—and, in particular, "self-sympathizing," "self-accusing," and "self-justifying" states. What everyone *wants* to do, of course, is to shift out of unpleasant (e.g., "self-accusing") states of mind and into pleasant (e.g., "self-sympathetic") ones. Unfortunately, we have only limited control of our states.

> We can try to talk ourselves out of a negative state of mind (a depressed or "self-accusing" mood) by reminding ourselves, for example, that others are worse off than we are and that we should be grateful for what we have.
>
> We can try to talk ourselves out of such a state of mind by appealing to cultural sayings.
>
> We can call up friends who we know are likely to be sympathetic, and avoid friends who we know are likely to be *un*sympathetic.
>
> We can do things that we hope will shift us into a pleasant state of mind, or at least distract us from unpleasant ones—go to a movie, for example, bake a cake, or take a bike ride.

These efforts are only partly successful, however. To the extent that we are *un*able to shift into pleasant ("non-self-accusing") states of mind, we need a backup plan. And my backup plan is to establish a vantage point—a platform—from which we can sympathize with ourselves for how life is a series of states of mind over which we have only limited control.

And that brings us to a major idea of this book: the platform.

PART 2

IMPLICATIONS FOR THERAPY: THE PLATFORM

I have described how Marie ratchets through alternative possibilities, snaps through states of mind, and struggles with self-blame. My goal, were I to see her in therapy, would be to enable her to *monitor* this ever-changing internal landscape rather than to be swallowed up in it. She needs a *platform*—a nonaccusing and nonanxious vantage point—from which to do this monitoring.

That is the heart of my therapeutic approach: to create such a platform. In Chapters 7 and 8, I describe how I try to do this. But first, in Chapter 6, I show how the therapist slips on and off his or her own platform.

The Therapist's Platform

Let us say that the day after the evening I have described in Part 1, Marie comes to see me for her weekly therapy session. (Paul is in therapy also, but he is seeing another therapist.) She tells me:

> I can't stand myself sometimes. I spent all last evening being this needy, demanding cliché of a wife. I stood in the kitchen like a dunce, unable to tell Paul anything. I hate evenings like that. My whole *day* was like that. I didn't have the guts to tell off my boss. And I didn't have the guts to tell off Paul. I'm a total mouse. And Jeannie and Billy were just horrible yesterday. They must be picking up the tension between Paul and me. Not only am I screwing up my life, I'm screwing up theirs. I don't know, maybe I'm just expecting too much of myself: having a family and a full-time job. But other women seem to manage. And I certainly shouldn't be stuffing myself with junk food.

As Marie continues in this vein, I have the following internal conversation:

> Marie is clearly upset with herself—her harsh internal taskmaster has taken over—but I am not sure yet how to talk with her about it.
> I wonder what Carl Rogers would do. Probably what he always does: sit on the edge of his chair and beam acceptance—like he did in that film with Gloria. That would be good, but whenever I act like Carl Rogers, it comes out phony. And, anyway, I'm after bigger game than self-acceptance.
> I know what Albert Ellis would do. He'd find an irrational idea and refute it. But what would he pick out here? Would he talk about

Marie's "awfulizing"? I'd better go back and read Ellis more carefully.

I know what Merton Gill (who focuses on making transference interpretations) would do: show Marie how she's really talking about her relationship with me. But what would he say *here*? Would he say she feels she's being a total mouse with *me*? Would he say she feels *I'm* being a total mouse with *her*? I should read Gill more thoroughly too.

I know what a strategic therapist would do: make a paradoxical intervention—maybe prescribe the symptom. I could tell Marie that if she *really* feels like a dunce, she could go the whole way and, tonight, wear a dunce's cap. I'm not one for paradox, but *that's* not bad. It might start a useful discussion between her and Paul.

I know what a cognitive-behaviorist would do: challenge Marie's negative self-talk. What a marvelous term—"negative self-talk." It really captures something. Whoever invented it deserves a medal. Who was it, anyway? Meichenbaum?

I know what Greenholtz, the behavior therapist down the hall, would do: give Marie a homework assignment. He is able to come up with one to fit any situation. But what would he come up with here? I can't imagine. I'll have to ask him.

I *don't* know what Milton Erickson would do. He almost always comes up with something that wouldn't occur to me. So I might as well not even try to think about it.

I know what Alice Eberheart, the therapist on the radio, would do. She'd try to find out what Marie is getting out of her behavior—what the payoff is. But it's hard to imagine what possible payoff there is, since Marie seems so clearly miserable. Eberheart might say that Marie *enjoys* being miserable.

I know what my barber would do. He'd tell Marie, "Aren't you being a little hard on yourself?", and hope that would snap her out of it. That's chancy. Marie is likely to take it as a reproach—that she *shouldn't* be so hard on herself. That's how I react when my barber says such things to me. Anyway, I want Marie to learn something about her self-accusation—not just snap out of it.

I know what Farland, the therapist across town, would do. She'd try to figure out what it was in Marie's childhood that led to such behavior. She'd ask Marie who "being like a total mouse" reminds her of—and expect Marie to say "my mother" or "my father." Maybe that's what *I* should do too—childhood *is* pretty important. Of course, what's most crucial for Farland is how clients *get to be* the way they are, whereas what's most crucial for me is how clients *feel about*—and *deal with*—the way they are.

So while I listen to Marie, I run through this series of thoughts, just as Marie, the night before, has run through her own series of thoughts.

And, just as Marie has snapped through various states of mind, this morning I have snapped through my own. The two sessions I had just prior to this one with Marie did not go well—which snapped me into the "feeling-not-so-great-as-a-therapist" state.

And on my way to pick up Marie from the waiting room, I ran into Greenholtz (the therapist down the hall), who told me about a success he just had with a homework assignment he gave a client. This snapped me into the "self-reproaching, maybe-I'm-shortchanging-my-clients, maybe-*I*-should-be-giving-homework-assignments-too" state.

And while I ushered Marie into my office, I began to think that it is not just homework assignments, but a whole set of techniques and approaches that I ought to be using—which snapped me into the "self-reproaching, I'm-too-committed-to-one-approach, maybe-I-should-look-at-all-the-other-approaches-and-see-what-they-have-to-offer" state.

In fact, it is because I am in this state that, while listening to Marie, I ratchet through these various therapeutic approaches—Rogers's, Greenholtz's, Farland's, and the rest.

> Thinking of what all these other therapists might do is making me dizzy.
> It's making it hard for me to focus on what *I'd* want to do.
> What *would* I want to do? I don't know.
> Of course, if I were my old supervisor, Casterhazen, I'd know what to do. I'd have figured out something brilliant to say.
> Casterhazen is remarkable.
> *He* should be seeing Marie instead of me.

Comparing myself to Casterhazen saps what remains of my self-confidence. I snap into the "self-reproaching, Marie's-unlucky-to-be-seeing-me, she-should-be-seeing-Casterhazen" state. And being in this state, I become a somewhat less attentive and somewhat less effective therapist:

> I'm not listening to what Marie is saying very well.
> I'm having difficulty *concentrating*—in fact, I just missed Marie's last two sentences completely.
> I feel disconnected from Marie.
> And *I'm* beginning to crave a chocolate donut.

Ordinarily, I might consider the possibility that my difficulty understanding, concentrating, and feeling connected is, at least in part, a response to what Marie is doing. But to be able to think about it this way—that is, to use my countertransference feelings as a clue rather than simply criticize myself for having them—I would have to be in the "feel-ing-okay-as-a-therapist" state of mind, which, of course, at the moment I am not.

But is my reaction typical? What about therapists who do *not* ratchet through alternatives, snap through states of mind, and feel inadequate? Well, actually, most of the time, I am such a therapist myself. My ratcheting, snapping, and feeling inadequate typically occur as an unnoticeable background buzz, bursting into the foreground only occasionally.

And what brings them into the foreground? Circumstances such as those I have just described: a run of sessions that do not go well; events that stimulate thoughts and feelings (e.g., anger, boredom, confusion—each therapist has his or her own particular set) that temporarily undermine my therapeutic self-confidence. Therapists who do not have (or at least are unaware of) the kind of thoughts I have just described handle their feelings in other ways. They drift off and, for example, think about their next vacation. Or they come away from the session feeling a little down without knowing why.

But what about therapists who *are* aware of such background thoughts (self-talk), but not of *self-accusing* ones (*negative* self-talk)? As I see it, these therapists do have self-accusing thoughts, but they snap through them very *fast* (too fast to register) and focus instead on the corrective or compensatory reactions. In fact, if I were in a different mood, I might do that myself. I might skip through my "Casterhazen-should-be-seeing-Marie-instead-of-me, self-reproachful" thought and focus instead on the time in supervision when I was able to point out something that Casterhazen missed. Then, instead of being distracted by the thought "Marie's unlucky to be seeing me, she should be seeing Casterhazen," I would be distracted by the thought, "Wasn't that a brilliant thing I said that time to Casterhazen?"

Here is my point: My capacities as a therapist come and go—and the same holds true, I believe, for every therapist. Being the kind of therapist I want to be requires being in a particular state of mind, which no one can be in all the time.

I have this platform from which to notice how my capacities come and go. And that partly protects me from always expecting myself to function at an optimal level and then getting upset with myself when I don't. I am in a good position if I am able to accept that there will be moments when I am going to:

Get distracted and be unable to use my countertransference reactions as clues.

Drift off; fade out; lose my ability to think, listen, generate ideas—
or even *remember* therapeutic principles that in other states of
mind are second nature to me.

Become bogged down in self-critical thoughts and be unable to be
the kind of therapist I want to be.

And I am having such a moment now:

I'm not understanding what's going on very well; I'm having difficulty concentrating; and I feel disconnected from Marie.

Clearly something is wrong with my empathy. Jeffrey Masson (interviewed in Beneke, 1988) says the best therapists are warm older
women. Maybe Marie should be seeing a warm older woman.

Listen to me. I'm as caught up in negative self-talk as Marie is. How
can I possibly be of help to her? We *both* need Carl Rogers or
Casterhazen or a cognitive-behavior therapist or Jeffrey Masson's
warm older woman.

So, as I sit listening to Marie, who is being invaded by her harsh
internal taskmaster, I am being invaded by mine. But whereas Marie's
harsh internal taskmaster attacks her with *cultural* sayings ("You have
no guts," "You're this total mouse," "You're screwing up your kids"),
mine attacks me with *professional* sayings:

You're failing to empathize.

You're narcissistic or, worse, schizoid—you're so disconnected from
Marie that you can't even listen to what she's saying.

You've got too many problems yourself to be able to be a therapist.
You're one of those therapists who went into the field to solve
his own problems.

You should go back for more therapy.

You're not cut out to be a therapist—you should have gone into
administration.

Your countertransference is getting in the way.

You're doing *dis*therapy. You're doing what Marie's father did to her
long ago and what Paul does to her now: You're withdrawing from
her.

Am I really this hard on myself—simply for having had two inconclusive therapy sessions before seeing Marie, for comparing myself to
Greenholtz and Casterhazen unfavorably, and for momentarily becoming a little inattentive?

Yes.

My purpose in this book is to put a microscope to the moment-to-moment experience of both the client and the therapist: to slow it down, magnify it, and expose all the half-thoughts and half-feelings that generally go unnoticed; that is, to reveal the self-talk that goes on in all of us.

Another therapist might react in a different way, of course. *I* might react in a different way if I were in a different mood or had gone to a different graduate school, had had different supervisors or a different therapist, had seen Marie earlier in my career when my approach was somewhat different, or had a different theory.

If I had a different theory, I might have reacted to the two inconclusive therapy hours I had with the clients I saw before Marie (a drifting session with Greg followed by a confusing one with Emily), and to my concern that I might be having the same kind of unsatisfactory hour with Marie:

> By adopting the "don't-get-discouraged, plod-on-and-hope-for-the-best" stance. I would tell myself, "Therapy is a vague and uncertain enterprise. You can never tell what is going to help the client or what the client might get from what you say. Anyway, it's probably not *what* you say that counts; it's the relationship you develop with your clients."
>
> Or by adopting the "don't-get-impatient, therapy-takes-a-long-time" stance. I would tell myself, "It took 20 or more years for Greg, Emily, and Marie to develop their problems. It might take just as long to resolve them."
>
> Or by adopting the "they're-resisting" or the "they're-seriously-disturbed" stance. I would tell myself, "Greg is unable to open up; he's unwilling to give up his anger. And what can I expect of Emily, anyway? She's borderline. As for Marie, she's . . ."
>
> Or by adopting a "the-problem-is-the-mode-of-therapy" stance. I would tell myself, "It was a mistake for me to go along with Greg's request to drop down to every other week. I should have stuck to my guns and insisted on seeing Marie in couples therapy rather than individual therapy. As for Emily, she should probably be seeing a female therapist."
>
> Or by adopting the "blaming-the-referral-source" stance. I would tell myself, "All three of them got my name from the Hendrick Clinic. This is the *last* time I accept referrals from them."

By the same token, if I had a different theory or a different character, or were in a different mood, I might have reacted in one of the following ways to Greenholtz's telling me about his successful homework assignment:

By telling him a success story of my own. That is, I would adopt the "let's-exchange-success-stories" stance.

Or by telling Greenholtz how his story immediately made me feel that I have been doing therapy all wrong—I should start giving homework assignments to all my clients. That is, I would adopt the "confiding-in-him-about-my-envy" stance. By expressing my envy, I would not be so weighted down and controlled by it.

Or by reminding myself of the clients who did not like Greenholtz and came to see me. That is, I would adopt the "dealing-with-the-story-by-privately-taking-him-down-a-peg" stance.

Or by telling Greenholtz that he jumped in too quickly to try to solve the client's problem, rather than developing further understanding of it; that he eliminated the symptom but not the cause, and there is going to be symptom substitution; or that he is dealing with the copper of suggestion rather than the pure gold of analysis. That is, I would adopt the "do-you-think-that-giving-that-assignment-was-really-such-a-good-idea?" stance.

Or by reminding myself that each therapist develops a sense for certain approaches and techniques. Giving homework assignments is one of Greenholtz's but it is not one of mine. That is, I would adopt the "each-therapist-has-his-or-her-own-particular-approach" stance.

But, instead of any of these, I adopted the "taking-it-as-a-personal-failure, the-problem-is-me, I'm-shortchanging-my-clients" stance. So now what do I do?

Well, I do not just sit there and take it. I defend myself. I *counter* my harsh internal taskmaster's admonishing professional sayings with professional sayings of my own:

A Battle of Sayings

MY TASKMASTER: You're having a failure of empathy.

ME: Failures of empathy are inevitable in psychotherapy, and, if Kohut (1984) is right, may even be part of the curative process.

MY TASKMASTER: You're narcissistic. That's why you're having difficulty listening to what Marie is saying, and that's why you feel disconnected from her.

ME: Maybe *Marie* is narcissistic. Maybe *that's* why I'm having difficulty listening to her and why I feel disconnected from her.

MY TASKMASTER: You've got too many problems yourself to be able to help Marie with hers.

ME: My problems or lack of them isn't relevant.

MY TASKMASTER: You should go back for more therapy.

ME: I can't go back for more therapy every time I hit a snag.

MY TASKMASTER: You're unsuited to be a therapist. Have you ever thought of going into administration?

ME: It's not a matter of temperament—psychotherapy is something that can be learned.

MY TASKMASTER: Your countertransference is getting in the way of the therapy.

ME: My countertransference is how I *do* therapy. It is how I figure out what is going on. It is one of the major ways I pick up how Marie feels about me, about herself, and about the therapy.

MY TASKMASTER: You're doing *dis*therapy. You're doing to Marie what her father did to her long ago and what Paul does to her now: You're withdrawing from her.

ME: Maybe Marie *wants* me to withdraw from her. Maybe she *wants* me to be distracted and to feel disconnected from her. She may have set up the whole thing—unconsciously. Whatever I do and feel is what Marie *wants* me to do or feel. My feelings are the result of her projective identification.

For some therapists, the idea that Marie may have unconsciously set up the whole thing is the heart of the matter. Given their theory, it is what they would come up with first. It is how these therapists think when they are at their best; that is, when they are *not* distracted by self-accusation or other countertransference factors.

When *I* have this idea, it means that I have gone off the deep end. It is how I think when I am at my worst; that is, when I am overwhelmed by self-accusation or other countertransference factors. Because this idea is so foreign to my thinking, I immediately jettison it:

> That's ridiculous. Look at Marie. She'd love some help. She doesn't want me to withdraw. What could I possibly be thinking of?

So these are the thoughts and feelings that go through my head as I sit there, saying nothing, listening to Marie. As Meichenbaum (1991) said in describing a session, "I talked the whole hour and I even said some things to the client." I have been talking the whole hour too, but I have yet to say anything to Marie. My talking has taken the form of an ongoing conversation with myself:

> *About myself* and, in particular, about the kind of therapist I am—
> "Am I a good therapist (in which case Marie is lucky to be seeing

me) or a poor therapist (in which case she's unlucky to be seeing me)?"

About my relationship with Marie—"Why am I having difficulty concentrating on what Marie is saying? Why do I feel disconnected from her?"

About other therapists and their theories—"What would Rogers, Ellis, Gill, Erickson, Greenholtz, and Casterhazen do in this situation? Am I shortchanging Marie by not giving her homework assignments or by not asking more about her childhood?"

About my theory—"What would *I* ordinarily do in this situation?"

With all these conversations going on, how can I think? Of course, that is what much of "thinking" is: such voices.

Yes, but how can I think *objectively*? How can I even hear what Marie is saying with all these layers of insistent voices making conflicting demands? At the moment, not very easily.

Fortunately, these voices typically exist as barely audible background sounds blaring out only for brief moments—although, of course, with some clients and in some sessions, they blare out constantly. And I have already begun to come out of it. Some of the sayings with which I have countered my harsh internal taskmaster's sayings take hold—that is, I begin to believe them:

Maybe my reactions are clues to what is going on rather than just indications of personal defects.

Maybe my inability to listen to Marie and my feeling of being disconnected from her *aren't* entirely my fault.

Maybe I'm having trouble listening because Marie is talking in an unengaged way. And *of course* she is. Her thinking is blocked; she's going around in circles.

And maybe I feel disconnected from Marie because she feels disconnected from me. And, now that I think of it, *of course* she must feel that way. She's caught up in worries and self-reproaches. She feels hopeless, and she probably doesn't see how I can possibly help.

Poor Marie.

And suddenly I am feeling sympathetic toward Marie. A major point in this chapter is that our capacities as therapists (e.g., our abilities to think, listen, generate ideas, draw upon our psychotherapeutic knowledge, and use our countertransference feelings as clues) come and go. They require being in the right state of mind. The same is true of our capacity to empathize with our clients. It is hard to feel sympathy or empathy toward others when we are under siege from our harsh internal taskmasters ourselves—that is, when we are in "self-accusing, non-self-sympathetic" states of mind. At such a moment, we shift into the "back-against-the-wall, pulling-the-wagons-around-us" mode, which leaves little room for concern about anyone else.

But, at the moment, I am in the "sympathizing-with-Marie" mode. My realization that my difficulty listening to Marie is a consequence of what *she* is doing—and, in particular, her relating to me in a closed-off way—allows me to get the blame off myself. I snap out of my "back-against-the-wall, unable-to-feel-concern-for-anyone-else" position and feel sympathy for Marie. In other words, getting the blame off myself—although the effect is to put it onto Marie—allows me to sympathize with her:

> Poor Marie—for having her thinking blocked, and for having all these self-reproaches.
> And poor me—for having my *own* thinking blocked, and for having *my* self-reproaches.
> I always feel bad when I'm unable to listen well—I think I'm not doing my job.
> And I always feel bad when I think how much more skillful Casterhazen is—which makes it even harder for me to listen well.
> So I'm really caught.
> What a shame that life has to be this way.
> I wonder if Casterhazen ever has such problems. I wonder if he ever gets discouraged when comparing himself to his own mentors. Lucky Freud—being the first therapist, he didn't have any mentors.

A shift has taken place. For a moment at least, I am no longer anxiously rattling through possibilities, snapping into dysphoric states of mind, and struggling with self-blame. I am no longer telling myself, "What's wrong with me for feeling the way I do?" Instead of blaming myself, I am sympathizing with myself. I am telling myself, "It's too bad I feel the way I do."

I am on the platform. Being able to sympathize with myself for the situation I am in is the criterion for being on the platform. It is how I *know* I am on it.

Now, you might wonder how Marie and I are to have any sort of useful conversation with all the ratcheting, catapulting, and self-blaming we are doing. Well, that is where the platform comes in. That is the ultimate answer to my harsh internal taskmaster's question: "How can I possibly help Marie when I have problems of my own?" That is the edge

I need to be able to help Marie. That is what I need if I am to do more than just muddle through. I need a platform from which to monitor my own ratcheting, catapulting, and self-accusing.

How does a platform help? The more I am on the platform—that is, the more I take my distractedness, envy of Greenholtz and Casterhazen, blame of Marie, self-reproach, and so on as a matter of course rather than as a sign that something is wrong with me:

> The less distracted I will be by them.
> The less I will have to struggle against my reactions.
> The more I will be able to use my reactions as clues.
> The more I will be able to sympathize with Marie.
> The better I will be able to listen to her.
> The more I will be able to generate ideas and draw upon my psychotherapeutic knowledge.
> The better I will be able to help Marie create a platform of her own.

That is the major task of therapy: helping clients create a platform. And it is the task to which I now turn.

CHAPTER 7

The Client's Platform

My goal in therapy is to create for Marie the same kind of platform that I have just created for myself. In fact, that is the heart of my therapeutic approach. Here is what I say to myself:

> I'm snapping back and forth between self-reproach and having a perspective on it. But it looks like Marie is *not*. It looks like she is just caught up in hers.
> So, let's see if I can think of something that might reveal whether Marie has a perspective on her self-reproach and, if she doesn't, that might give her such a perspective.

Here is what I say to Marie:

So, you're not particularly happy with yourself at the moment.

It may seem like a lot of thinking (i.e., everything I have described in the preceding chapter) to yield such an ordinary intervention: a simple Rogerian reflection. But this is often the amount of thinking that goes into even the most banal comment. Although it is a simple Rogerian reflection, I expect a lot more from it than Rogers did. Rogers wanted to give the client the experience of being received, heard, and totally accepted. He wanted to provide an atmosphere of unconditional positive regard. I want that too. But I want something more: I want to bump Marie up a level. I want to create a "non-self-reproaching" vantage point—a platform—from which she can look at her self-reproach.

Unfortunately, I am not securely on my *own* platform—which makes it difficult for me to help Marie create hers. I am experiencing the residue effects of unfavorably comparing myself to Greenholtz and Caster-

hazen, and of those inconclusive hours with the two clients I saw earlier in the day; that is, I have not fully regained my capacities as a therapist. Were I to regain them, I would be able to say to Marie, "It sounds
as if you are in the state of mind we talked about last time—in which
you hate yourself but don't know it because you're so deeply in it."
Instead, I express a more tentative thought: "So, you're not particularly
happy with yourself at the moment."

And Marie reacts to my tentativeness:

> Happy? How can I be happy when I waste the entire evening stand-
> ing in the kitchen like a dunce, filling my face with potato chips?

Marie is saying, in effect, "I feel all this distress, and the best you
can say is 'You're not particularly happy with yourself at the moment.'
You must be a dunce not to know that I feel like a dunce. You haven't
a *clue* to what I really feel." Sensing that Marie is saying that, I snap
into the "feeling-I've-said-the-wrong-thing, feeling-all-the-more-that-I'm-
not-a-very-good-therapist" state. Not only have I failed to get Marie on
her platform, but I have fallen off mine. I struggle on:

> Okay, so you felt bad about the way you behaved.

Halfway through this sentence, I realize that this intervention has
the same problem. It, too, understates Marie's feelings. If I could suck
the words back into my mouth, I would. I hope that Marie will not notice
them—or at least that she will let them pass.

Not a chance. She replies:

> *Of course* I felt bad about the way I behaved. You'd feel bad too if
> you spent the whole night feeling sorry for yourself and eating
> like a pig.

Marie's "Of course" is short for "Of course, you dummy; don't you
understand anything?"

THERAPIST: You seem impatient with me.
MARIE: I'm *not* impatient. I'm just saying that there was absolutely no
  excuse for my behaving the way I did last night.

Marie appears to have taken my "You seem impatient with me" as
an accusation—as meaning "You *shouldn't* be impatient with me." And
she is right to do so. That *is* what I meant—although I didn't know it at
the time. A communication skills trainer might point out that my comment "You seem impatient with me" is a "you statement" and, in addi-

tion, "mind reading." My countertransference is showing; I am retaliating for Marie's shortness with me. Instead of a platform—a *non*accusing vantage point from which to look at what she is doing—I have created an *anti*platform: an *accusing* vantage point.

When I hear myself saying, "You seem a little impatient with me," my alarms go off. I snap into the "unhappy-with-myself, oh-oh, what-am-I-doing?, I'm-violating-one-of-my-major-principles" state of mind.

I know that the intervention "You seem a little impatient with me" may seem to many therapists useful and to the point. If Marie does feel impatient with me, after all, it does seem important to talk about it. In fact, this intervention is one of the more benign in a whole range of common therapist comments; less benign examples include "You seem angry at me," "You're leaving me out," "You're being defensive," and "You're trying to control the hour."

The problem with such interventions is that it is hard for people to hear them without thinking that they are being rebuked, or without at least *wondering* whether the therapist is disapproving of them. And when clients feel rebuked, they generally become angry, self-accusing, defensive, or withdrawn, or in some other way lose the ability to think. (Wachtel, 1993, has recently described the subtle ways in which therapists become rebuking without realizing it.)

I try to avoid this problem by making clear that I am *not* rebuking my clients—by saying, for example, "It's *understandable* you might feel impatient with me," "It *makes sense* that you might want to leave me out," or "*Anyone* might get defensive in such a situation."

In saying to Marie, "You seem impatient with me," I am violating this principle. I am *not* making it clear that I do not mean this as a rebuke. Fortunately, I have a "self-forgiving, non-self-accusing" vantage place from which to spot myself making this error. In fact, I feel clever and skillful for being able to spot it—and for knowing how to correct it. I respond to Marie's objection ("I'm *not* impatient. I'm just saying that there was absolutely no excuse for my behaving the way I did last night") by saying:

THERAPIST: Well, actually, you've been really clear about that—so you must feel I'm being a little dense *not* to get it.
MARIE (*smiles*): Well, maybe just a little.

I have gotten Marie on the platform. She and I are sympathizing with her for the situation she is in—even if this situation is having a therapist (me) who she feels is not listening to her and with whom, accordingly, she has reason to feel impatient:

THERAPIST: Well, okay, if I *am* being dense, let me try to see what I would see if I *weren't* being dense. I'd say that you felt *terrible* about how you behaved last night, that you saw it as totally unacceptable—that it set you back *years*. Well, I don't know about that part—I just made that up—I don't know if you felt it set you back *years*. But, anyway, it really demoralized you. You saw it as inexcusable. And then what *I* said might have sounded as if I were trying to give you an excuse, or saying it *wasn't* so bad, or failing to appreciate how terrible you felt about it.

MARIE: *Now* you've got it. In fact, you said it even better than I did. I *especially* liked the part about how "it set me back years." Except you underestimated— it set me back *decades*. I haven't behaved like that since I was a shy little 5-year-old girl—although, of course, *Paul* didn't help any; he behaved like a selfish little 5-year-old boy. He buried himself in the living room. He forgot that someone else lives there too. And I wasn't even asking for that much: just a little participation in our home life. But *no*. Right away he disappears to watch the News. He doesn't want to hear *my* news.

It is easy to miss—since it happens so quickly—but Marie has just snapped from the "blaming-myself" to the "blaming-Paul" state of mind.

What do I do? What I *want* to do is create a platform from which Marie can view this shift. So I say:

Now *that's* interesting. Just a second ago you were blaming yourself. Now you're blaming Paul.

And even while I say this, I sense something amiss. If I had time to think about it, I would realize that I am trying to force Marie onto the platform. I am trying to get her to look at how she is blaming Paul before she has finished the blaming—in fact, before she has hardly begun it. I am trying to force her to be objective before she has finished being non-objective. We each press our points:

MARIE: *Of course* I'm blaming Paul. He was a total creep. You should have seen the way he dashed into the living room—like a rat through a hole in the wall.

THERAPIST: Yes, well, *that's* what's so interesting. You're seeing Paul as a rat. And a moment ago you were thinking of yourself as a rat or, rather, as a mouse.

MARIE: That's exactly it. I'm the mouse—you know, sweet, cute, cuddly, something you'd want to hold. Paul's the rat. He disappears down the rat hole, never to be seen again.

Why is Marie not joining me in looking at how she has just snapped from the "blaming-myself" to the "blaming-Paul" state. Why is she refusing to get on the platform? Because in her present state of mind, she has no interest in the platform. Instead, she is expressing her frustration. She is getting the blame off herself by giving it to Paul. And that is something I ought to appreciate; just a few moments ago, I was getting the blame off myself by giving it to Marie.

Marie and I are talking past each other. *I* am trying to get her to notice that she has just shifted from the "blaming-myself" to the "blaming-Paul" state, and *she* is trying to prove that Paul deserves to be blamed. So I try to create a "not-talking-past-each-other" vantage point from which Marie and I can *notice* that we are talking past each other. I stop trying to make *my* point. Instead, I come over to her side and help her make hers:

THERAPIST: Well, I've been pressing this point about how you shifted from blaming yourself to blaming Paul. But maybe I should listen to what *you're* saying. And what you're saying is that Paul forgets that someone else lives in the house and that someone is you. He disappears through a hole in the wall. He plops down in front of the TV and won't even speak to you. He's interested in news about the world, but he doesn't want to hear your news—news that should matter to him too. So, putting that all together, you must be feeling—what is it? Rejected? Neglected? Dismissed? Isolated?

MARIE: Well, more than *any* of those things: I feel *abandoned*.

THERAPIST: Of course—abandoned.

MARIE: I hate it when Paul runs away to watch the News. I feel deserted—and then I go a little crazy. I see him as totally responsible for all our problems . . .

There is an edge to Marie's tone—a touch of anger—which means that she is *not* on the platform. It is possible, however, that she is on the *verge* of being on the platform, since she is to some extent *reporting* her blaming state ("I *see* him as totally responsible") rather than just being in it ("Paul *is* totally responsible"). She is reporting on the circumstances that get her into that state (Paul's dashing away to watch the News). And she is reporting what it is like when she is *in* that state ("I hate it," "I feel deserted," "I go a little crazy," "I see him as totally responsible for all our problems"). To the extent that Marie is reporting being in the blaming state rather than just being in it—that is, to the extent that she is talking nonaccusingly about her accusations—she is on the platform.

A communication skills trainer might notice that Marie is making an "I statement." In fact, Marie's "When Paul does such-and-such, I feel such-and-such" is a classic form of "I statement." "Being on the platform" can be thought of as another way of talking about "I statements":

> It is a way of talking about "I statements," however, that reveals why "I statements" are so special—and why everyone recommends making them.
>
> It is a way of talking about "I statements" that reveals why the "Make 'I statements,' not 'you statements'" rule is difficult to obey. Shifting from a "you statement" to an "I statement"—if it is to be a *true* "I statement"— means snapping into a new state of mind. It means suddenly being on the platform. Simply mouthing the words "I feel such-and-such" will not do it.

To get back to Marie, it is not entirely clear at the moment whether or not she is on the platform—that is, whether she is simply *reporting* her "blaming-Paul" state—or whether she is still *in* it. She says that when Paul dashes away to watch the News, "I feel deserted, I go a little crazy, and I see him as totally responsible for all our problems . . ." She adds:

> . . . that is, of course, when I'm not seeing *myself* as totally responsible for all our problems.

To me, this means that Marie *is* firmly on the platform. She is reporting how she can shift between blaming Paul and blaming herself. And it means that I again have an opportunity to raise the issue that I have tried unsuccessfully to raise before:

THERAPIST: Yes. Well, actually, earlier in the hour you made such a shift from seeing yourself as totally responsible to seeing Paul as totally responsible.

MARIE: Hmm. I guess I did.

Encouraged by Marie's willingness to go along with what I just said, I press on:

THERAPIST: What do you think might have led to that shift?

MARIE: I don't know.

I try to stimulate Marie's thinking on the matter by getting her back into the situation:

THERAPIST: Well, let's recreate the scene and see if we can figure it out. You came in feeling bad—you saw yourself as this little mouse who retreated to the kitchen and ate chips. Then I said something that made you feel that I didn't appreciate how horrible you felt about it. Then you described yourself as this "shy little 5-year-old girl." I think it was at *that* point that you made the shift: You said that Paul was this "selfish little 5-year-old boy."

MARIE: You left out the *important* part.

THERAPIST: What was that?

MARIE: The part when you said that it set me back years.

THERAPIST: Okay, so *that* was the turning point.

MARIE: I didn't feel so alone.

THERAPIST: Alone?

MARIE: Yes, that was the problem—I felt alone with Paul last night. And I felt alone with you this morning—until you said that thing about it setting me back years.

THERAPIST: How did my saying that make you feel less alone?

MARIE: I felt you understood, which was really different from the moment before, when I felt that you *didn't* understand. But then I got this longing feeling.

THERAPIST: Longing?

MARIE: You'd given me a taste of what it's *possible* to get—but that just made me aware of what I ordinarily *don't* get.

THERAPIST: Which is—?

MARIE: What I got from you—you know, someone who . . . Maybe you were out of tune with me—but it was possible to bring you *in* tune.

THERAPIST: Okay, so someone who's—

MARIE: And suddenly I got furious at Paul for *not* being in tune with me, for not even *trying* to be in tune—for disappearing into the News instead of staying with me and making the effort.

Marie has found what we both have been looking for—the explanation for her shift from blaming herself to blaming Paul. But I am not sure that she has realized what we have discovered. That is my job—to keep tabs on what we are discussing, to remember what we are doing, to point out when we have discovered what we have been looking for:

THERAPIST: Okay, so *that's* what led to your shift from blaming yourself to blaming Paul. The moment of understanding you got from me made you aware what you don't get from Paul—and you got angry just thinking about it.

MARIE: Maybe I just expect too much. Paul works hard all day at the store. I shouldn't begrudge him a little escape.

With these words, Marie slips off the platform and back into the self-accusing state in which she feels unentitled to her feelings and wishes. It is my job to keep track of this too:

THERAPIST: Well, it sounds as if you might just now have shifted to blaming yourself.
MARIE: Maybe I shouldn't have blamed Paul in the *first* place.
He doesn't have to be a rat to want to escape into the News.
THERAPIST: But you still could *wish* that he'd listen, instead, to *your* news. You still could *wish* that he'd come into the kitchen, look you in the eye—or, better, put his arms around you—and say that he wanted to hear what had happened to *you* today.
MARIE: Wish! I'd fall over in a faint. But I can't *expect* him to do that.

Marie has snapped into the "obligation-oriented, what's-okay-and-what's-not-okay-for-me-to-expect" state, in which the world is defined in terms of duties, responsibilities, and role expectations. When she is in this state, there is no place for wishes. (She feels unentitled to wishes.) Wishes cannot coexist with obligations—they are wiped out by them. She temporarily loses the concept "wish."

So I want to create a platform from which Marie can realize that she is *in* the "obligation-oriented" state in which there is no place for wishes. In reply to her "But I *can't* expect him to do that [i.e., turn off the TV and listen to my news]," I say:

THERAPIST: But you could still *wish* he would.
MARIE: I don't have the right.
THERAPIST: How come?
MARIE: Well, I don't know . . . it's just that . . . well, actually—I don't know . . . I'm confused.

I want to challenge Marie's idea that she does not have a right to her wishes. But first I am going to have to help her state this idea:

THERAPIST: Well, let's see if I can help you get *un*confused. You're saying that you shouldn't expect more from Paul than you feel you have a *right* to expect from him.
MARIE: Yes. He works hard all day—he has the right to watch the News.
THERAPIST: And then you're saying that even just *wishing* that he would

listen instead to your news turns you into a person who expects more than she has a right to expect.

MARIE: I know it sounds ridiculous.

THERAPIST: And the ridiculous part is—?

MARIE: It sounds so horribly self-sacrificing—I'm being such a martyr.

I have successfully challenged Marie's idea that she does not have a right to her wishes. It is easy to miss that I've done this, however, because she immediately transforms it into a renewed self-reproach. She has snapped from the "I-don't-have-a-right-to-my-wishes" stance to the "I-*do*-have-a-right-to-my-wishes, there's-something-wrong-with-me-for-thinking-I-don't, I-must-be-a-martyr" stance.

THERAPIST: Well, it's clear that you don't like this picture we've just drawn of you.

MARIE: Of course I don't like it. I don't want to be a martyr. *No one* wants to be a martyr.

"Martyr" is one of those terms—"lazy," "irresponsible," "selfish," "codependent," "workaholic," "wimp," and "nag" are others—that are judgments in the guise of descriptions. They are stop-you-in-your-tracks put-downs that bring an end to useful thinking about the matter. I try to undo Marie's self-reproach so that we can resume thinking.

THERAPIST: Maybe we need a "martyr's liberation movement," just like we need a feminist movement and all the other liberation movements.

MARIE: What do you mean?

THERAPIST: Well, when you say that you're "being a martyr," you—

MARIE: I mean that I'm too self-sacrificing, that I use it to control other people, and that I haven't the guts to stand up for my own rights.

THERAPIST: Well, if there *were* a "martyr's liberation movement," and if you belonged to it, you'd be appreciating what you're dealing with instead of just seeing yourself as dealing with things "wrong."

MARIE: But I do appreciate what I'm dealing with.

THERAPIST: I don't think so—because if you did, you'd see yourself as suffering an acute form of every woman's problem: being expected, and expecting herself, to take care of others—to put other people's needs ahead of her own. And you'd see yourself, understandably, as uncertain about what you *can* expect from others. And you'd see yourself as, at times, getting satisfaction out of doing for others and dedicating yourself to their welfare—but understandably at other times rebelling against the whole thing and wondering when you're going to get your chance. And you'd think it a shame that, in addition to everything else, you have to get down on yourself for all of this—that you have to see yourself as a "martyr."

MARIE: Well, I still don't think I should need Paul to listen to my news after he's had a hard day.

This means that Marie has snapped back into the "obligation-oriented" state, in which she feels she does not have a right to her own wishes—or even her "needs."

MARIE (*continuing*): It's selfish—and it's unrealistic—because it's not going to happen. So there's no point in wishing for it.

THERAPIST: Oh, are you saying then, "Why wish for something when it's not going to happen and so I'm only going to be disappointed? It's better not to wish for it in the first place"?

MARIE: Yes. Why get my hopes up?

THERAPIST: Of course, I imagine it's hard *not* to get your hopes up.

MARIE: I know. I can't seem to stop wishing that Paul *would* want to talk to me more—even though I know that I shouldn't.

THERAPIST: I'm not surprised.

MARIE: You're not?

THERAPIST: It's hard to *stop* yourself from wishing for things.

MARIE: What do you mean?

THERAPIST: Wishes are hard to turn off—everyone just has them. And you can't choose what they're going to be.

MARIE: Hmm.

THERAPIST: So there's Paul, and he's having *his* wishes—he's wishing that you would leave him alone, or that you would do all kinds of wonderful things for him, or that he would win a million dollars, or that they make him manager of the store.

MARIE: Well, I *know* he's wishing I'd leave him alone—and, maybe also that they promote him to manager.

THERAPIST: Okay, so he's having those wishes. And you're having *your* wishes, which would include that Paul turn off the TV, come into the kitchen, and listen to *your* news.

MARIE: But what good does wishing do? It's not going to happen.

Marie has again scooted on past me. She has snapped out of the "obligation-oriented" stance and in and out of the "self-sympathetic; okay, maybe-I-am-entitled-to-my-wishes" stance, coming to rest back in the "why-get-my-hopes-up-only-to-be-disappointed" stance. I try to trace the "zig-zag, particle-in-physics-passing-through-a-bubble-chamber, all-happening-in-a-fraction-of-a-second" path of her thoughts:

THERAPIST: So you're saying, "Okay, sure, everyone's got their wishes—and I've got my wishes. I wish that Paul would come into the kitchen and listen to my news. *But*, it's not going to happen—Paul's not going to do it—so I might as well not get my hopes up."

MARIE: You got it.

THERAPIST: So you're feeling *discouraged*.

MARIE: *More* than just discouraged—hopeless.

THERAPIST: Hopeless?

If Farland were in my office observing the session, she would hardly be able to contain herself, wanting me to ask Marie: "With whom have you had such a feeling of hopelessness before?" Farland, as I have noted in Chapter 6, is the therapist across town who traces everything to childhood. She would want me to get to what she sees as the heart of the matter—to go back to the early growing-up years, where the action is.

Of course, if Farland were the therapist and I were the observer, *I* would hardly be able to contain myself, wanting Farland to shift from focusing on the origin of Marie's feelings in childhood to focusing on how Marie is managing those feelings *now*. I would want Farland to get to what I see as the heart of the matter, where the action is— *the platform*. I would want her to focus on the relationship Marie is having with herself *about* her childhood-caused sense of hopelessness. I would want Farland to direct attention to how able Marie is to do the following:

Think about, feel about, and deal with her feelings of hopelessness and abandonment.

Relate to herself as a person who has such feelings.

Plan for these feelings to recur, as opposed to hoping they won't recur—in fact, *counting* on them not to recur—and being unprepared when they do.

Become an expert in dealing with them.

Appeal to others as resources for dealing with them.

Have an ongoing conversation with herself (and with Paul) about these feelings.

Make these feelings part of her relationship with Paul and part of her relationship with herself.

I would want to construct a theory with Marie about her recurrent feelings of hopelessness and abandonment—that is, to create a platform from which she could notice, keep an eye on, be curious about, and deal with these feelings.

If, as I said, Farland were the therapist and I were the observer, I would want Farland to talk with Marie about how Marie is relating to her feelings. But I would also admire what Farland would be accomplishing by devoting therapy to tracing her feelings to childhood. Farland would be helping Marie discover the ways in which her feelings toward Paul are holdovers from her experiences with her father long ago. Marie felt that her father continually let her down. He broke promises to her. He made plans to spend time with her and then cancelled them. Despite assurances to the contrary, he did not show up for her senior class play, in which she had a major role. She felt she could not count on him—just as she feels she cannot count on Paul.

True, I would get to this material in my own way—although not as quickly and systematically as Farland, and not in such detail. And I would miss certain important parts. Every therapeutic approach enables a therapist to detect certain important things and causes him or her to miss others.

Fortunately, Marie had previously consulted Farland; she saw her about problems with her daughter, Jeannie. Both Marie and I are thus now able to profit from Farland's childhood-oriented approach. In our exploration of her feeling of "hopelessness," Marie remembers something that came up in her sessions with Farland:

MARIE: I must have been 8. My father promised to pick me up after school and show me where he worked. But he never showed up. And I stood on the corner shivering in the cold.
THERAPIST: Hmm.
MARIE: You know—last night with Paul—it's funny, but standing in the kitchen, I got this little chill.
THERAPIST: As if you were 8 years old back on the corner?
MARIE: Yes. And I had to put on my sweater—even though I was working in the kitchen and it was hot.

If Greenholtz, the behavior therapist down the hall, were observing this session, he would hardly be able to contain himself, wanting to make sure that I would not spend the entire hour analyzing the problem without even *beginning* to help Marie figure out what to do about it. If Greenholtz were conducting the session, he would start making therapeutic suggestions much earlier, when Marie was criticizing herself for standing in the kitchen like a mouse. He would recommend that Marie follow Paul to the living room and talk to him. He would give Marie assertiveness training or communication skills training, and send her home with an assignment to practice these skills.

Of course, if Greenholtz were the therapist and I were the observer, *I* would hardly be able to contain myself, wanting Greenholtz to stop his suggestions, skills training, and homework assignments, and instead to focus on how Marie was *managing* her feelings. But I would also be aware that Marie might benefit from the suggestions and the skills training. And, at some point, I, too, would want to bring up the possibility of Marie's going into the living room and talking to Paul:

THERAPIST: Okay, there you were last night—feeling alone, abandoned, and hopeless; getting this chill; feeling almost like you were back there waiting for your father; feeling like a mouse. Let's look at that for a moment. What does a person *do* in such a situation?

MARIE: I don't know. You're supposed to tell me.

THERAPIST: Right. But let me ask you anyway. Let's say that it wasn't you, but a friend of yours who was in the kitchen feeling what you were feeling last night. And *she* comes to *you* and tells you all about it. What would you say to her?

MARIE: That she should talk to her husband about it.

THERAPIST: Okay, let's say you're *you* now, and your friend's your friend—and that's the advice she gives you. What would you think of that advice?

MARIE: I'd think of it as useful—but I wouldn't follow it.

THERAPIST: Why not?

MARIE: I wouldn't know what to *say* to Paul.

THERAPIST: How about what you just said here, to me? You'd go into the living room and you'd say, "You know, standing in the kitchen just now, I got this chill—almost as if I were back on the corner waiting for my father when I was 8. Except I wasn't feeling it about my father—I was feeling it about *you*. Things got off on the wrong foot tonight, and I didn't know what to do about it. So I was just standing there, feeling alone, afraid to come in and tell you all this—and feeling upset with myself for being such a mouse."

MARIE: Paul would be shocked—he'd never expect to hear anything like that from me. I'd be shocked myself.

THERAPIST: Do you *like* the idea of saying it? Is it something that you would have said if you'd thought of it?

MARIE: I wish I *had* thought of it.

THERAPIST: How do you think Paul would respond if you *were* to say it?

MARIE: He'd say, "I'm *tired* of having to pay for what your father did."

Therapist: And, hearing him say that, you'd feel—?

MARIE: I'd say, "Listen, I came in here to try to make things better. I was reaching out. And what do you do? You take advantage of it to get in a dig. You're *always* doing that. There's no way to talk to you about anything."

THERAPIST: And then what would happen?

MARIE: Paul would scowl, I'd stomp out, and he'd give me the silent treatment.

THERAPIST: Then—

MARIE: Then, when he'd finally say something, I'd give *him* the silent treatment—and I'd be sorry I came out of the kitchen at all. If I'd stayed there we wouldn't have had the same silence, and we'd have saved ourselves all those awful words.

If Greenholtz were the therapist, he would try to think of what Marie could say that might rescue the conversation. I might too. But first I would point out to Marie that what she has just said shows us why she behaved the way she did last night. It makes sense of it. It explains it. It allows us to sympathize with her for the dilemma she was in:

THERAPIST: Well, maybe *that's* why you *did* stay in the kitchen "like a mouse": because *not* being one—going out and talking to Paul— seemed worse to you.

MARIE: Hmm, maybe so.

THERAPIST: So, you were really in a fix. No wonder you went for the potato chips.

Why do I interrupt the important task at hand—helping Marie figure out what she could have said that might have rescued the conversation—to help explain why she behaved the way she did last night? *Because it is not what Marie says to Paul, but what she says to herself that is crucial.* The conversation that Marie has with herself is the important one. My goal is to tap into this conversation, to make it explicit, to reveal its reproachful nature, and to give her a glimpse of a non-self-reproachful alternative:

THERAPIST: Okay, so we now have a different picture than the one you had when you first came in today.

MARIE: I don't see the difference.

THERAPIST: Well, when you first came in, you said there was no excuse for sitting in the kitchen like a mouse and nibbling chips. But now we're saying there *is* an excuse—or at least an explanation. We're saying: Oh, so *that's* why you sat in the kitchen—because you felt that the alternative, going out and talking to Paul, would have been worse. And *that's* why you went for the chips—because you needed *something*. And the *major* difference between the picture you had of yourself when you first came in and the one we have of you now is that we're sympathizing rather than blaming you for the difficult situation you were in last night.

MARIE: Can I take you home with me? I really need someone who can think like that for me.

What am I doing here? The same thing I have been doing throughout the hour: trying to give Marie a glimpse of what the world would look like from a nonaccusing vantage point. What I have just said for her is what she herself might say if she were already on the platform.

The platform is always my central concept. Whatever else I do— whether it is discussing what Marie might have said to Paul, tracing her problems to childhood, exploring options, analyzing the transference, analyzing the countertransference, whatever—my focus is on creating a platform.

I believe that many therapists are groping for what I call "the platform"—and that they know when they have found it. It is unmistakable. It has the ring of "Yes, that's the perspective I want to have" and "Yes, that's the perspective I want my clients to have." As it stands now, however, the platform is part of our "back-of-the-mind, no-one-ever-told-us-about-it, we-had-to-figure-it-out-for-ourselves," informal knowledge that we apply in a hit-or-miss fashion.

In the next chapter, I show how it might look if we were to recognize the platform as the active ingredient and organizing element of our therapeutic approach.

CHAPTER 8

The Value of the Platform

Everyone is always on the verge of being overwhelmed by his or her feelings—or losing track of them—and we need a perspective from which to monitor all of this.

Even before a client walks into my office, I already know what his or her problem is: the lack of a platform. How do I know this? In the same way that Ellis knows that the problem is irrational beliefs and that Freud knew that the problem was an Oedipal conflict. I assume it. It is the unprovable—and un*dis*provable—idea I start with.

How does this focus on "the platform" affect my therapeutic work? As you may remember, Marie begins the hour by saying:

> I spent all last evening being this needy, demanding cliché of a wife. I stood in the kitchen like a dunce, unable to tell Paul anything. I hate evenings like that. My whole *day* was like that. I didn't have the guts to tell off my boss. And I didn't have the guts to tell off Paul. I'm a total mouse.

As I listen to Marie, I make a simultaneous translation. I imagine what she might say if she were on the platform:

> I've been spinning like a top because of what happened last night. I'm really upset with myself. And I've been looking forward to coming here; I felt I wouldn't feel so alone if I could tell you about it. And what's astonishing is that it's exactly what we were talking about last time—you know, how I can really get down on myself. Except I figured out something new. The *main* thing I get down on myself for is "being a mouse"—having no guts. Now *being* a mouse is problem enough, so it's a shame that I have to make it even harder for myself by beating myself up for it. And I real-

ized something else. Not only do I criticize myself for what women criticize themselves for—being a nag and a martyr; I also criticize myself for what *men* criticize themselves for—having no guts and being a wimp. I don't like seeing myself as a nag, a martyr, and a wimp, so I try not to think about it. I just grit my teeth and try not to be these things. But maybe it's good to think about these things, because that's what I'm doing right now and it helps; I've stopped spinning around. And I can even sympathize with myself, at least for the moment, for having all these things to deal with.

How would this alternative version of Marie's report reveal that she is on a platform?

1. Marie would be bringing me in on what she wants from me ("I've been spinning like a top because of what happened last night. I'm really upset with myself. And I've been looking forward to coming here; I felt I wouldn't feel so alone if I could tell you about it").

2. She would be *curious* about the problem so that figuring something out would be exciting ("And what's astonishing . . .").

3. She would be having an *ongoing* conversation with herself, and with me, about it (". . . it's exactly what we were talking about last time— you know, how I can really get down on myself").

4. The conversation would be a *developing* one ("Except I figured out something new. The *main* thing I get down on myself for is 'being a mouse'—having no guts").

5. She would be sympathizing with herself, being her own confidant, being a one-person consciousness-raising group for discovering and dealing with her prejudices against herself ("Now, *being* a mouse is problem enough, so it's a shame that I have to make it even harder for myself by beating myself up for it").

6. She would be sitting with the problem. That is, she would be able to really think about the problem and feel the feelings associated with it, rather than immediately having to solve it or, failing that, having to deny that it *is* a problem, resign herself to it, or just avoid it ("I don't like seeing myself as a nag, a martyr, and a wimp, so I try not to think about it. I just grit my teeth and try not to be these things. But maybe it's good to think about these things, because that's what I'm doing right now and it helps; I've stopped spinning around").

7. She would be creating a new, nonanxious, nonaccusing relationship with herself about the problem, and *that* is the solution ("And I can even sympathize with myself, at least for the moment, for all these things I have to deal with").

The platform offers an *overview position*—Marie would have bumped herself up a level. She would have a *new and self-sympathetic attitude* toward the problem and toward herself for having it. As a result of this new attitude, Marie would be able to "have" the problem—that is, to sit with it, inhabit it, really think about it.

When people talk about "sitting with a problem," they generally mean becoming mired in it, going around in circles, being unable or unwilling to take constructive action, being a "Hamlet." And indeed that is what sitting with the problem can mean when you are *not* on the platform. When you are *on* the platform, it means having new thoughts, discovering new feelings, developing new information, and making new discoveries. It means becoming increasingly expert in monitoring, planning for, and recovering from the problem.

Creating Moment-to-Moment Platforms

At any given moment in a session with Marie, I try to imagine what Marie might say to herself if she were on the platform. And I try to find a way to bring her in on what I am imagining—and to get *her* interested in the task of building such a platform. To show how I do this, I shall go back over the therapy excerpt I have just described in Chapters 6 and 7, focusing this time on how, from moment to moment, I try to create a platform.

When, at the beginning of this excerpt, Marie criticizes herself for "being such a mouse," I try to give her a sympathetic view of how she is being self-accusing; that is, I try to bring her in on the "view-from-the-platform" statement that I am imagining for her. Unfortunately, what I say ("So, you're not particularly happy with yourself at the moment") makes her feel that I am minimizing the problem—that is, not taking seriously how upset she is.

This means that Marie now has a *new* experience—feeling she has a therapist who is not "getting it"—which is now my task to help her view from the platform. And here I am more successful. I tell her, "You must feel I'm being a little dense *not* to get it." For a moment Marie and I are on the platform, sympathizing with her for having a therapist she feels is not in tune with her.

But just for a moment—since almost immediately Marie begins blaming Paul. Her feeling that I finally *am* in tune with her only makes her aware that Paul *never* is in tune with her—and she gets angry at him. So Marie is now having yet another new experience—blaming Paul—which is now my task to help her view from the platform. And, after several false starts, I succeed. For a moment Marie and I are back on the platform, this time noticing that she is blaming Paul.

But just for a moment, since Marie almost immediately shifts to blaming herself for blaming Paul (she feels she should not begrudge Paul wanting to watch the News) and then into an "obligation-oriented, not-having-a-right-to-my-wishes" state of mind—which is now my task to help her view from the platform. I describe how wishes are inevitable—everyone has them—and that one of hers was that Paul come into the kitchen last night and listen to *her* news. For a second Marie has a "nonanxious, nonaccusing" vantage point from which to look at this wish.

But just for a second, since Marie immediately begins to feel discouraged about Paul's ever satisfying it. And it is now Marie's "feeling-discouraged, feeling-hopeless" experience that I want to help her view from the platform. But this time Marie takes the initiative. She traces her feelings of hopelessness to her relationship with her father long ago. She remembers the time when she waited for him in the cold and he never showed up. "You know—last night with Paul—it's funny," she says, "but standing in the kitchen, I got this little chill."

This means that this new experience—the "sympathizing-with-myself-for-having-such-a-father" experience—is now the one I want to help her view from the platform. I could say, "It's a good thing you're able to blame your father, in view of all the difficulty you've had with that." I don't do this, however, because I am not thinking fast enough.

And that is too bad, because Marie is in *particular* need of a "non-self-accusing" vantage point from which to look at her accusing of others. Since she feels uncomfortable about being accusatory (particularly toward her father), she does so in a grim, rigid, and defensive manner.

As I see it, "being on the platform" includes appreciating the ways in which your behavior may be an understandable reaction to the present situation—independent of any ways in which it may also be an understandable consequence of your childhood.

With this in mind, I try to discover ways in which Marie's behavior last night may be an understandable reaction to what she had to deal with at the time. I try to help her appreciate her no-win situation: She could stand in the kitchen and feel like a timid mouse, or go into the living room to talk to Paul and get into a fight. For a moment—and in response to my comment—Marie has a "nonaccusing, self-sympathetic" vantage point from which to look at her dilemma. She is on the platform.

This is what I try to do with clients—provide moment-to-moment platforms throughout the session. Whatever Marie is concerned about or engaged in at the moment, I try to create a platform from which she can look at it. And whatever Marie is concerned about or engaged in the *next* moment, I try to create a platform for that.

But how is this going to help Marie?

MARIE: I don't see how any of this is going to help me.

THERAPIST: Well, it *would* help if, for example, the next time you find yourself feeling like a mouse, you remember some of the things we just talked about. You wouldn't be stuck, as you were last night, with just the one thought, "I'm this *bad* person." You'd have *other* thoughts. You'd think, "It's a *shame* that I see myself as a bad person." Or you'd think, "I can *see* why I see myself as a bad person: That's what happens when I feel alone and abandoned—I blame myself." Or you'd think, "I'm not this *bad* person; I'm this *unfortunate* person—I'm in a no-win situation, caught between feeling like a coward and getting into a disagreeable argument."

MARIE: Yes, but—

THERAPIST (*too caught up in the point to notice she has an objection*): And the next time Paul disappears to watch the News and you feel abandoned, you wouldn't be stuck with just the one thought, "I *shouldn't* resent it; Paul has a right to watch the News." You'd now have the *new* thought, "But I still could *wish* that Paul would listen to my news," and be *disappointed* that he doesn't.

MARIE: Yes, but—

THERAPIST: And the next time you see yourself as a martyr, you wouldn't be stuck with just the one thought, "I'm this horrible person—a martyr." You'd now have the *new* thought, "It's too bad that after all this time seeing it as my *job* to sacrifice for others, I suddenly turn on myself and accuse myself of being a martyr."

MARIE (*finally getting the therapist's attention*): Well, yes, all that's very nice—but I'm not going to be *able* to tell myself those things. Not any of them. I'm not even going to remember them. In fact, I'd already forgotten them—I needed to hear what you just said to remind me.

Marie has a point here (now that I've stopped talking long enough to allow her to make it). These ideas are hard to remember. They don't stick in the mind. They're too foreign. They don't fit into familiar categories. And many of them are counterintuitive. They fly in the face of what Marie already "knows":

> How is Marie going to remember that she sits in the kitchen feeling like a mouse because she is in a no-win situation? That flies too much in the face of what Marie "knows," which is that it is "weak" when she doesn't pursue what she wants.
>
> And how is Marie going to remember that it is okay to wish that Paul would listen to her news? That flies too much in the face of

what she "knows," which is that she "should just learn to accept things the way they are; she shouldn't try to change people."

And how is Marie going to remember the "martyr's liberation movement"? That flies too much in the face of what Marie "knows," which is that it is "bad" to be a martyr.

If Marie is to remember these things, or anything else I have discussed with her, she has to be in the right state of mind:

In order for Marie to realize that she felt abandoned by Paul last night, she has to be in the "feeling-sympathized-with-by-my-therapist" state of mind.

In order for Marie to feel angry at Paul, she has to be in the "feeling-I-am-getting-something-from-my-therapist" state of mind so she can appreciate—and sympathize with herself for—what she is not getting from Paul.

In order for Marie to be able to have the objectivity and presence of mind to figure out why she gets angry at Paul (or in order for her even to be interested in figuring it out), she has to be *over* her anger with him; that is, she has to be *out* of the "blaming-Paul, hating-Paul" state of mind.

Now we can see why therapy is so difficult. Therapy requires making available to the client certain ideas and feelings that are:

• Unfamiliar—they do not fit in with what is already in the client's mind.
• Counterintuitive—they *contradict* what is in the client's mind.
• Or momentarily irretrievable—they are locked away in states of mind to which the client lacks immediate access. Horowitz (1987) and Ornstein (1989) describe how certain ideas are available only in certain states of mind.

The therapeutic task is to make these unavailable ideas and feelings accessible. One way to do so is to give clients glimpses of them, as I try to give Marie a glimpse of the idea of a "martyr's liberation movement" and the idea that "everyone has a right to his or her wishes."

Often I am unsuccessful in giving clients this glimpse. Marie finds my discussion of "martyr's liberation" unconvincing. And when I am successful—Marie does suddenly get a glimpse of what it would be like if she were to feel she had a right to her wishes—the glimpse is often short-lived. Marie immediately snaps into the "feeling-discouraged-because-Paul-isn't-going-to-satisfy-these-wishes" state of mind.

So, given all these problems, why do I remain dedicated to creating platforms? Because I have no choice. Just as Albert Ellis, given his theory, has no choice but to dispute his clients' irrational beliefs; and Joseph Wolpe, given his theory, has no choice but to carry out systematic desensitization; and Carl Rogers, given his theory, had no choice but to engage in reflective listening; so I, given my theory, have no choice but to try to create platforms.

I want to give Marie glimpses of the platform:

First, to show her that such a thing exists, *despite* its being unfamiliar, counterintuitive, or momentarily irretrievable.
Second, in the hopes that she will increasingly be able to incorporate elements of the platform into her own thinking.

Creating a Permanent Platform

Throughout the session, I create moment-to-moment platforms. My goal is to enable Marie to create such moment-to-moment platforms for herself. But another goal is to create a *permanent* platform that Marie and I can refer back to and build upon—with the goal of enabling Marie to create such a platform for herself. So when, later in the hour, Marie says:

I feel a little better than when I first came in today—but just a *little* better—because I'm still upset that I sat in the kitchen last night like a scared little mouse completely unable to do anything.

—I take advantage of her comment to bring up an issue that we had been observing from the permanent platform: the "what-I'm-coming-to-therapy-for-and-what-we're-working-on" issue.

THERAPIST: Well, I'm not surprised because—though I know we haven't called it this before—isn't that what we've been talking about all along: your feeling of being a mouse? In fact, isn't that what you originally came in about? I remember your saying in the first session that you felt "depressed, scared, and paralyzed."
MARIE: I don't think I'm *ever* going to change. I don't even think it's *possible* to change.

Marie is caught up in the "feeling-hopeless, I'll-never-change" state of mind. So, in this next statement, I remind her how, at other times, she is able to view this feeling from the permanent platform.

THERAPIST: There's that feeling of hopelessness that, as we've begun to get good at noticing lately, can rush in suddenly and take over.

And now I bring up another idea that we have been observing from the permanent platform: "are-we-accomplishing-what-we've-set-out-to-accomplish, is-therapy-really-helping?":

THERAPIST (*continuing*): I can see why it did so just now. We've been working on the "scared-mouse" feeling, in one form or another, for some time without clear progress. And you've been working on it by *yourself* even longer.

MARIE: My whole life.

I am trying to create a *permanent* vantage point from which Marie and I can monitor, among other things, what is happening in therapy, why she is coming to therapy, and what she is getting from the therapy. And I do this because:

The reasons for which clients come to therapy evolve, change, and clarify over time. It is important, therefore, to update our knowledge continually.

Therapy is an experiment to see whether talking to a therapist (or at least to *this* therapist) is useful. It is important, therefore, to evaluate periodically whether therapy *is* useful—that is, whether it is worthwhile to continue.

Therapy is a joint management effort. It is important, therefore, to have a forum in which to exercise this joint management. Lynn Hoffman talks about "putting the client on the board of directors" (interviewed in Simon, 1992, p. 164).

Therapy, as I see it, is the learning by clients of a new way of thinking about themselves and their reactions. It is important, therefore, for clients to be able to talk about what they are learning in order to solidify this new way of thinking and to discuss their doubts about it—that is, whether it makes sense to them.

Therapy is, in part, an inquiry into what is concerning the client at any given moment, with the assumption that such discussion will shed light on the major issues for which he or she is coming to therapy. It is important at some point, therefore, to tie in what we discover in a given session with these major issues.

As part of our developing understanding of what Marie is coming to therapy for, I ask:

THERAPIST: Okay, now that we've got this new way of talking about what you're coming in about—the "scared-little-mouse" feeling—what more can you say about it?

MARIE: I conk out.

THERAPIST: You mean—?

MARIE: It's like I suddenly lose 50 IQ points. My mind goes blank. I can't think of anything to say. It's like I'm paralyzed. When I told this to Dr. Farland, she thought I might have been sexually abused by my father.

Immediately I snap into the "did-I-miss-the-signs-of-incest? am-I-one-of-those-unenlightened-male-therapists-who's-insensitive-to-women's-issues?" state of mind:

THERAPIST: What did you tell her when she said that?

MARIE: That I remembered the *opposite*—that my father didn't seem very interested in me, or at least he kept disappointing me. And my mother never did anything about it when he disappointed or ignored me. It was like she wasn't all that interested either.

THERAPIST: And what did Dr. Farland say?

MARIE: That we still should keep an eye on the possibility that he abused me.

THERAPIST: And what did you think about that?

MARIE: I could see her point—but I still didn't think that anything like that ever happened.

THERAPIST: And how do you feel about it now?

MARIE: The same way.

Since Marie sounds sufficiently convincing about this for the moment, I return to the point I have been developing:

THERAPIST: Okay, so there you are in the kitchen, feeling like a mouse, getting a chill, feeling you're back on the corner waiting for your father, losing 50 IQ points, unable to think of anything to say, feeling paralyzed.

MARIE: I hate it when I get like that.

THERAPIST: And what you *most* hate about it is—?

MARIE: I don't know—well, it's so "weak." It's the way my mother was sometimes.

Hearing Marie refer again to her mother, I snap into the "Farland-might-be-right, maybe-I-should-focus-even-more-than-I-do-on-tracing-problems-to-childhood" stance.

THERAPIST: Okay, so you—

MARIE: It rules my life. If I see myself as a timid mouse, the way I did last night, it ruins me—there's no recovery. I lose every shred of self-respect. If I *don't* see myself as a timid mouse, then I'm okay.

Wonderful! I feel that Marie may have latched on to something really crucial here. She says that feeling like a timid mouse rules her life—it determines whether on any given day she feels okay about herself. If this turns out to be true, then Marie has given us a powerful tool. She has updated (i.e., added an important new wrinkle to) the "timid-mouse" idea from the permanent platform. From now on, Marie and I can look at her days through the clarifying filter of whether or not she feels like a timid mouse.

I have snapped out of the "self-critical, Farland-might-be-right, maybe-I-should-direct-even-more-attention-to-tracking-problems-to-child-hood" stance and into the "self-reassuring, I-should-learn-not-to-doubt-myself, it-makes-sense-to-focus-therapy-on-building-a-permanent-plat-form, using-childhood-as-a-means-to-this-end" stance.

THERAPIST: That's quite a discovery—that whether you get into the "timid-mouse" state determines whether the day is ruined. Is that an idea that you're speculating about and aren't quite sure of? Or is it something that really seems right?

MARIE: It really seems right.

THERAPIST: Did you just figure it out now, or is it something that you've known all along?

MARIE: Well, I've *sort* of known it all along—but this is the first time I've put it into words.

THERAPIST: Am I the only one getting excited about it, or does it seem pretty important to you, too?

MARIE: It's pretty important.

The fact that Marie agrees that it is pretty important does not necessarily mean that she is going to remember it. That is *my* job—to remember such things, to be guardian of the permanent platform—as a step toward making *her* guardian of it.

The Next Session

So it is no surprise that Marie comes to the next session and proceeds as if we had not talked about the "timid-mouse" feeling. She describes an incident with her boss.

THERAPIST: You seem unhappy with yourself this week in the same way you were last week.

MARIE: I don't remember last week.

THERAPIST: You criticized yourself for being a mouse.

MARIE: Oh, yes. Well, it's *exactly* the same this week. My boss called me into her office, and I just stood there tongue-tied while she criticized the memo I wrote to the finance department. Everyone else liked the way I really laid it on the line, but all *she* could think about was one little insignificant point that I left out. Only a mouse would put up with it.

THERAPIST: What would you have done if you *hadn't* put up with it—that is, if you *hadn't* been a mouse?

MARIE: I'd tell her that *she* was supposed to write that memo—I did *her* job—so she has some nerve criticizing it.

THERAPIST: And if you *were* to tell her that?

MARIE: She'd start a file on me. She'd try to get me fired.

THERAPIST: She *would*?

MARIE: I wouldn't put it past her. She started a file on Gerald for less.

THERAPIST: Well, if that's what you think would happen, maybe you're seeing yourself not so much as a *timid* mouse for keeping your mouth shut, as a *smart* mouse who wants to keep her job.

MARIE: It doesn't matter whether it's smart or dumb. I still feel it's weak. And it still ruins my day.

So now we have this further bit of information to add to the "feeling-like-a-timid-mouse-ruins-my-day" idea. As long as Marie feels it is "weak," it can ruin her day, even if acting like a mouse is, in her judgment, a wise thing to do.

And Subsequent Sessions

In my beginning years as a therapist, when clients came to a session and expressed difficulty starting (e.g., "I don't know what to say"), I made sure not to play into their "resistances," "pulls for dependency," or "fantasies about my enacting a magical cure." I turned it back on them by focusing on their difficulty. Yet I don't remember much useful coming out of it. At best they would stumble through it and, after a moment or two, get started. At worst, they would stumble the whole hour.

I had been taught that a client's difficulty getting started, like a client's cancelling appointments or coming late, was grist for the mill; it was a useful place to make therapeutic contact. My clinical experience, however, was that raising these issues often *clogged* the mill—that such issues were typically a poor place to make therapeutic contact. Clients felt that they were being *accused* of something. They thought they should not have trouble starting the hour, or come late, or miss appointments. When I directed attention to their trouble starting and so on, they grew contrite or defensive; that is, they snapped into states of mind in which it was impossible for them to think productively.

In recent years—now that the platform is my major therapeutic concept—I am often *happy* when clients have difficulty getting started, since that gives me an opportunity to bring up what I want to bring up: ideas from the permanent platform.

So when Marie comes to the next session and says:

> I don't know what to talk about today. Nothing much has happened this week.

—I first snap into my "remembering-what-I-learned-in-my-early-training" stance. I momentarily think, "Maybe I should ask Marie what lies behind her 'I don't know what to talk about today.'" Immediately I reject the idea, however, remembering the very modest benefits that were reaped the last hundred times I asked this question. Instead, I take advantage of Marie's hesitant beginning to bring up the "timid-mouse" idea from the permanent platform.

THERAPIST: Well, if you're not sure what you want to talk about, let me bring up something that I want to talk about.
MARIE: Good.
THERAPIST: I was struck the last two times with the "timid-mouse" idea. It really seems to capture something. So I wonder whether it struck you also—and whether you've had any further thoughts about it.
MARIE: It *did* strike me—though I haven't thought any more about it. I was too busy nursing Jeannie through the flu. And then I caught it from her and I was too busy being sick.

In order to be able to bring up this idea from the permanent platform, as I have just done, I have to be able to remember it—and, in fact, to have it at my fingertips. So I make an effort, in the note that I write following each session, to keep track of these platforms.

THERAPIST: What struck me particularly about last session was your idea that the day is ruined or not, depending on whether you get your "scared-mouse" feeling. What do you think about that now?
MARIE: It still seems right. In fact, that's what happened Saturday. I was a mouse, and it ruined everything I touched that day. I stayed home

nursing Jeannie through her flu, feeling sorry for myself, and resenting Paul's having a good time taking Billy to a baseball game.

THERAPIST: You didn't get to—

MARIE: What's worse is that it was my own choice—in fact, it was *my* idea that they go to the game. I thought it would be good for them to get out of the house. At first I felt okay about it—I don't even like baseball that much. But then I thought, "Why does Paul always get to go out? Why doesn't *he* ever stay home with the kids when they're sick?" And I got upset at myself for being such a martyr and for being so dumb—for not *knowing* I would end up resenting being left at home.

THERAPIST: You had a *way* of knowing?

MARIE: Well, actually, it was only when they stayed out later than I expected—the game went into extra innings—that I had trouble with it. Otherwise I might not have minded. In fact, I was worried enough about Jeannie that I wanted to stay home with her.

THERAPIST: So you felt all right about it at first—but then, when they were late getting back, it hit you another way.

MARIE: Yes, but I shouldn't have felt resentful.

THERAPIST: Why not?

MARIE: There wasn't any reason.

I snap into my "feminist-critique, noticing-how-Marie-gets-stuck-with-all-the-organizing" stance.

THERAPIST: Well, I don't know. Didn't you tell me that even though Paul does a lot around the house—more than most husbands you know—it's still *you* who has to do all the organizing and all the making sure that everything gets done? Maybe you tapped into that. You did say that it's always you who stays home when the kids are sick.

Marie: Well, actually, that reminds me of *another* time this week that I felt like a mouse. It was Paul's turn to do the vacuuming and he wasn't doing it—and I just stood there afraid to remind him.

Marie has scooted on to the next subject. It is *as if* she has said, "Okay, you've convinced me—maybe I *do* have a right to feel resentful about always having to take responsibility. But that reminds me of something else I wanted to tell you about—the vacuuming."

Immediately I snap into the "Marie-was-afraid-to-remind-Paul-that-it-was-his-turn-to-do-the-vacuuming, maybe-I-should-do-what-Greenholtz-would-do-and-give-her-assertiveness-training" stance.

THERAPIST: And what you were afraid of was—?

MARIE:—that, sure, if I made a point of it, he'd grab the vacuum cleaner
and do the rugs, but he'd stop talking to me. I was afraid I'd lose
him for the evening.

THERAPIST: Is that what usually happens?

MARIE: That's what *always* happens.

Once again we see how Marie became a mouse because she felt that
not becoming one would cause worse problems—in this case, she would
lose Paul for the evening.

So, that is how I try to create a permanent platform. My goal is to
make the ideas on this platform part of Marie's operating consciousness—
her working knowledge of herself. My ultimate goal, probably unachievable, is that Marie will be able to come into a session and say something like this:

> I've been thinking all this week about the "scared-little-mouse" feel-
> ing and how it controls my life. And I *watched* it control my life.
> On Tuesday I stood by while my boss unfairly criticized Gerald.
> I was feeling okay at the time, but I knew that just standing by
> like that was going to catch up with me. Sure enough, a little later
> I began to feel horrible. But at least I knew *why* I felt horrible—
> and that was a help. And at least I knew I'd be able to talk to Paul
> about it—and *that* was a help. So, by the time I got home, I wasn't
> feeling quite as rotten. You know, I hadn't realized it before, but
> pinning down why I feel bad is a real help. On Thursday, I felt
> wonderful—on the way home I rented a tape I thought the whole
> family would like, and got some popcorn to go with it. I felt
> wonderful because I *hadn't* been a mouse. I found a way to talk
> to my boss about her criticizing Gerald. And I've been feeling
> pretty good ever since—although I'm a little worried about what's
> going to happen tonight. Paul is supposed to have mailed his
> mother's birthday present—and ten to one he hasn't done it. And
> if it's true he hasn't, I'll probably sit there quietly rather than be
> a nag. You know, if I'm going to be my mousy self, I might as
> well make the most of it and stop on the way home tonight and
> get some really good cheese.

In talking about the "scared-mouse, ruined-day" idea in this manner, Marie would be:

- Bumping herself up a level—she would be standing back and talking about the situation she was in, rather than just talking from
  within it.

- Thinking about the problem—she would be holding an ongoing developing conversation with herself about the problem.
- Being her own confidant—she would be forming a one-person consciousness-raising group for dealing with being a person who has such a problem.
- Monitoring the problem—she would be noticing when it occurs and planning for its recurrence.
- Discovering new things about it—she would be realizing that pinning down why she feels bad can help.
- Having a new attitude toward the problem—she would be commiserating with herself about the problem, and even having a sense of humor about it ("If I'm going to be my mousy self, I might as well get some really good cheese").
- Appealing to Paul as a resource in dealing with the problem (or at least part of it)—she would be confiding in Paul about her feeling like a mouse with her boss. And, by bringing home the cheese (since he is likely to ask her why she bought it, and they might get into a conversation about it), she would at least in this indirect and hesitant way be appealing to Paul as a resource in dealing with her feeling like a mouse with him.

In effect, Marie would be having compassionate relationship with herself about the problem. She would have taken for her own this idea that she and I had been viewing from the permanent platform: the "scared-mouse, ruined-day" idea.

So that is my probably unachievable goal, that is, what I would *like* to happen: that Marie come into a session and be able to talk like that. But what *does* happen? What *does* Marie come in and talk about?

Well, she begins the next session by saying:

> I got impatient with Jeannie this morning. And it's funny, because ordinarily that would upset me—I don't think a mother should get impatient with her kids. But this time I told myself, "Maybe I just 'tapped into something' the way Wile talked about it last week."

At first I wonder whether Marie was confusing me with someone else, since I do not remember mentioning her "tapping into" anything. But then I remember saying that she might have "tapped into" her complaint that Paul doesn't take responsibility for things getting done around the house.

THERAPIST: How did thinking you "tapped into something" help?

MARIE: Well, it meant that there was a way of thinking about what I just did that made sense of it. I wasn't just an irritable person—I . . . tapped into something.

THERAPIST: And what you tapped into was—?

MARIE: My worry that Jeannie is getting to be the same shy, withdrawn kid that I was. Because that's what upset me this morning—Jeannie's telling me that she didn't want to play with the little girl across the street. It was scary—it was like me 30 years ago. The last thing Jeannie needs is a mother who gets upset with her when she's feeling shy. But it's hard for me to stand by and see her so timid and lonely.

Several sessions later, Marie says:

MARIE: You know, I've gotten a lot of mileage out of the "tapped-into-something" idea. Lots of times, when I begin to get upset with myself for what I'm feeling, I think maybe I just "tapped into something."

THERAPIST: And when you think that you've just "tapped into something" you think—what?

MARIE: Well, it's like a voice telling me that things aren't as bad as I think—that *I'm* not as bad as I think—that *everyone* has things they tap into, and here is one of mine. And, furthermore, that it's a shame I have to get down on myself for it.

Marie is using "tapped into something," a phrase I used in passing, to counteract her self-critical voice and, in addition, as material for building a platform.

THERAPIST: We've talked about your attacking voice that calls you things like "a bad mother" and a "timid mouse." But now it looks as if you also have a reassuring voice that—

MARIE: Well, actually, it's *your* voice. I hear *your* voice saying "you just tapped into something."

THERAPIST: Oh—

MARIE: And I know that isn't good. I *shouldn't* be hearing your voice reassuring me. I should be able to reassure myself.

If Bacon, one of my former supervisors, were behind a one-way mirror observing this therapy session, she would call me on the phone and tell me:

Marie is dependent, and you've got to be careful not to play into it. You don't want to limit therapy to a transference cure. She's merging with you, and you've got to be sure to establish clear

boundaries. You should tell her, "Yes, you're right; it is important to learn to reassure yourself rather than imagining me doing
it." Or, if you want to put it more tactfully, you could say, "Well,
we're *working* toward your eventually being able to reassure yourself."

If Talcot, another former supervisor, were behind the one-way mirror with Bacon, he would snatch the phone out of Bacon's hand and
tell me:

I disagree. I'd tell Marie, "If imagining my voice helps, wonderful—
whatever works."

If Cotton, a third supervisor, were behind the one-way mirror with
Bacon and Talcot, she would take her turn on the phone.

Marie's problem isn't merging or dependency, as Bacon just said,
but rather her *accusing* herself of merging and dependency. Look
at what Marie said. She said she *shouldn't* be hearing your voice
reassuring her. She said she *shouldn't* need you to reassure her.
That's not a person whose problem is dependency. That's a person who's hating herself for any sign of dependency. I'd want to
defend her against her self-hate. When she says that she should't
be using my voice to reassure herself, that she should be able to
reassure herself, I'd say, "Using my voice is a *way* to reassure yourself. It's hard for people at times to be able to reassure themselves.
Any way they can do it, more power to them. If using my voice
helps, fine. The only thing wrong with using my voice to reassure yourself is that *you* think there's something wrong with it.
And there's nothing wrong with that either—since it's easy, given
what everyone has always told us, to believe that we shouldn't
count on others to reassure us."

And if my mentor, Casterhazen, were behind the one-way mirror
with Bacon, Talcot, and Cotton, he would take his turn on the phone
and say:

After defending Marie against her self-hate, I'd want her to have the
added benefit of being in on this debate we're having here behind
the one-way mirror—at least to the extent that it's also a debate
that's going on in her own head. I'd want to show Marie, how,
for example, she may at some moments be a Bacon, criticizing
herself for using your voice to reassure her; how at other moments

she may be a Talcot, telling herself, "Whatever works"; and how at still other moments she may be a Cotton, telling herself, "It's too bad I have to criticize myself for using Wile's voice to reassure myself."

I have my former supervisors' voices going on in my head just as Marie has my voice going on in hers. I want to give Marie the advantage, *à la* Casterhazen, of being able to listen in on her struggles with her self-accusing voice. I want her at any moment to be able to bump herself up a level, where she can see her reactions. I want to give her the same view of herself and her situation that I have. I want Marie to have a picture of how she shifts among states of mind. So I do what I imagine Casterhazen would recommend. I talk with Marie about the following:

How she is in an ongoing struggle with a self-critical voice, just like everyone is.

How she has found a way, at some moments, to counter her self-critical voice with a reassuring voice, my voice, saying, "You just tapped into something."

That the reassuring effect can be destroyed by the thought, "I *shouldn't* be hearing your voice reassuring me; I should be able to reassure myself."

And how she may, at some moments, counteract this reasserted self-critical voice by again imagining my voice, perhaps this time saying something reassuring such as this: "There is nothing wrong with using my voice to reassure yourself."

And, in general, how she shifts between self-critical and reassuring inner voices.

And how there is nothing unusual about that, since everyone shifts between such voices.

And after I finish, Marie says:

Hmm.

I do not know whether this is a "hmm" of recognition ("Oh, yes, I see") or a "hmm" of doubt ("What *is* this man talking about?"). But the hour is up and it is too late to find out.

The following session, Marie returns to the "scared-little-mouse" issue:

I was standing there on a movie line when this obnoxious woman cut right in front and I couldn't say a word—not *one word*. I hate myself as much as I always did when I act like that old mouse. Although this time it was a little different because I was *watching* myself. First I told myself that I "just tapped into something," and then I criticized myself for using your voice to reassure me, and then I defended myself by saying, "What's wrong with using his voice?" I never realized before what a battle goes on in my head.

Marie has lifted herself up onto the platform.

THERAPIST: That was quite a job of tracking the struggle going on within yourself.
MARIE: It helped—I didn't feel quite so powerless.

So that is what I do in therapy: I try to give clients a glimpse of what the world would look like if they were on the platform—with the hope that such thinking will creep into their operating consciousness. I may construct a from-the-platform conversation Marie might have with Paul or, as I do later in this session, a from-the-platform conversation she might have with herself:

THERAPIST: Let's go back to that time, a few weeks ago, when you were standing in the kitchen hating yourself for being timid. But let's imagine now that you were to say to yourself: "What a shame this has to happen to me. The day is already a total disaster—everything's gone wrong—and I'd been hoping to talk to Paul so I could feel that at least he was on my side. But Paul won't talk to me. And now I'm not even on my *own* side any more, because I can't stand myself when I sit in the kitchen and act so passive. It reminds me too much of the shy, withdrawn little kid that I used to be—and that I'm afraid Jeannie is becoming. It taps into that. And it taps into that old feeling I have of standing on the corner, shivering, feeling abandoned, waiting for my father who never came. This is not a good time to be me. And this is not a good time to be Paul, either—because I know he feels bad when things go sour between us as they've been."
MARIE: I'd *never* be able to talk to myself like that.
THERAPIST: Would you *want* to?
MARIE: Of *course*. It's so forgiving. And it's so comforting. But I'll never be able to do it.

Marie is recognizing the essence of the platform, that is, that it is nonaccusatory and self-forgiving.

THERAPIST: Well, actually, you've already learned to talk to yourself like that. Remember—when you were on the movie line, you noticed the

battle going on in your head, and you were able to be self-forgiving about it.

MARIE: That *was* pretty good, wasn't it?

I have talked about platforms in these last three chapters in three
ways:

1. The platform that I establish for myself, from which I monitor
   how I gain and lose my capacities as a therapist.
2. The moment-by-moment platforms that I try to establish for the
   client throughout the session.
3. The relatively permanent platform that the client and I can refer
   back to and build upon—and whose establishment is the goal of
   therapy.

BLAMING YOUR PARTNER

In individual therapy, when clients get caught up in blaming themselves, my goal, as I have shown in Part 2, is to create a platform from which they can monitor it. But, as I now show, blaming oneself often leads to blaming others and, in particular, one's partner. So in *couples* therapy, when partners get caught up in blaming each other, my goal is to create a platform from which they can monitor *that*.

In Part 3, I show how blaming yourself leads to blaming your partner and how a frequent result is a fight. In Part 4, I show how I deal therapeutically with fighting couples.

When last seen at the end of Part 1, Marie is in the kitchen making dinner, eating potato chips, and feeling bad. Now, her 7-year-old son Billy wanders in. What Marie talks about with Billy leads to a chain of feelings that gets her out of the kitchen, where she has been blaming herself, and into the living room, where she starts blaming Paul (Chapter 9). Paul sorts through 44 possible defensive responses (Chapter 10) and picks one, which leads to a fight (Chapters 11 and 12).

Blaming:
If You Can't Join Them, Beat Them

The shift from blaming yourself to blaming your partner is more complex than people generally realize.

Marie is standing by the sink, a crumpled bag of potato chips in one hand and a peeled onion in the other, when Billy, who just an hour ago was crayoning the walls, comes in and asks:

Mommy, will you read me a story?

She cannot believe it. Billy knows that she is not feeling kindly toward him. He knows that even if she *were*, she couldn't possibly read him a story while cooking. Talk about childish self-centeredness!

She is about to snap, "Not now, Billy. Can't you see I'm making dinner? Why don't you ask your father to read to you?" But suddenly Marie realizes that it is precisely *because* she is annoyed with him that Billy is asking her to read to him. He is trying to make amends. He is saying he feels okay about her, despite the fact that she yelled at him earlier. And he hopes she feels okay about him. He is looking for reassurance. He does not really expect to be read to; he just wants a friendly response.

Marie is charmed by his reaching out to her—he looks really sweet. So she gives him a big hug and says:

Sure, I'd love to read to you. Choose your favorite book and I'll read to you after dinner.

Billy's smile makes it clear that he has gotten the friendly response he came for.

But what a responsibility! Look at the cleverness and intuition it takes for Marie to figure out what Billy wants. She is not going to be able to do that all the time—she is lucky to be able to do it *this* time. Things happen too fast. Before she has time to figure anything out, usually something else happens that she also doesn't have time to figure out. And even if she has the time, she probably won't be able to figure it out—relationships are that subtle.

A point of this book is to slow things down, at least for this one evening. And the first thing we figure out is how overmatched Marie is—but how, nevertheless, at moments such as Billy's coming into the kitchen to ask her to read to him, she can momentarily see what is going on.

If Marie could take a moment to stand back and to appreciate what she just did with Billy, she would notice an irony. In asking Marie to read to him, Billy has reached out to her—just as earlier, in telling Paul about the difficulties of her day, Marie reached out to Paul. Except, somehow, Billy has done a better job than Marie did in reaching out. Or was it that she did a better job than Paul did in recognizing that she was being reached out to?

Here is how Marie thinks about the matter (although probably not exactly in these words):

> Billy's a wonderful kid—coming right out and asking me to read to him like that. And I'm pretty terrific too, the way I figured out what he really wanted. Not everyone could have done that.

Marie is proud of how she responded to Billy; it snaps her into her "self-appreciating, feeling-like-a-good-mother" state of mind. When she is in this state of mind, she feels that she is a deserving person. And feeling that she deserves something, she becomes aware of what she is missing. She tells herself:

> I want Paul to *want* to listen, and really be interested, when I tell him about days like this.

Snapping into her "self-appreciating" state of mind means suddenly becoming aware of wishes that, in her "self-blaming" state of mind, Marie does not feel she has a right to and does not know she has. She rushes into the living room to tell Paul about her wish. But when she opens her mouth, what comes out instead is this:

> You never talk to me any more.

Marie has gone into the living room to tell Paul a wish—and, instead, she makes a complaint.

What has happened? Well, in the few seconds that it takes to get there, Marie has another of the "happening-too-fast-to-be-completely-aware-of" internal conversations that we all have:

How nice it would be if Paul would understand me and reassure me, the way I did with Billy just now.

But isn't it childish of me to want that? Billy's 7 years old—I'm an adult.

And do I deserve it? I really screwed up today—letting my boss get to me, yelling at the kids, and the pigging out.

I saw Paul's look when he disappeared to watch TV. He doesn't want to have anything to do with me.

And I don't blame him. I'm overbearing and smothering. Why would *anyone* want to have anything to do with me?

Of course, I'm always willing to talk to him when *he's* had a bad day.

He owes me. He *should* talk to me.

A husband should talk to his wife, not withdraw into his cave while she slaves over his dinner.

And I know what he's going to do when I tell him I want him to listen to me. He'll *pretend* to listen, but he'll keep sneaking looks at the screen. And I'll say, "You're not listening." And he'll say, "Yes, I am. You were telling me about the kids and about your boss and . . ." And I'll say, "Yeah, you were listening, but you weren't *hearing*—you weren't really *interested*." And he'll say, "Yes, I was."

And if I persist, he'll say, "Can't this wait until later? I'm in the middle of the News."

And that would be fine, except that he's not going to want to talk later either.

Why can't he be like my girlfriends? It's so easy to talk to them.

He's ruining my marriage.

These thoughts flash by too quickly for Marie to register them fully. All she knows is that when she reaches the living room and opens her mouth, what comes out is "You never talk to me any more." Her doubt that Paul will listen to her—combined with her feeling that she doesn't have the right to ask him to—has turned into indignation at his unwillingness to fulfill what Marie now sees as his *duty* to her.

Marie has snapped into a state of mind in which she sees Paul as the source of her problems—as unconcerned about her welfare and working against it. She has shifted into the "blaming-Paul, hating-Paul, Paul-is-the-source-of-my-problems" state of mind.

This new state of mind is so different from the one Marie has just been in that it is hard to believe that Marie is the same woman. And, in a way, she is not the same woman. There are several Maries, and several relationships she is having with Paul. She can tell when she has just shifted to a new relationship with him because she suddenly feels different—and Paul looks different. These states that Marie shifts into and out of last for seconds, minutes, or hours.

A Short List of Different Relationships
That Marie Is Having with Paul

Tense with Paul: nervous, careful, inhibited, tentative, walking on eggshells, watching what she says, worried about starting a fight or hurting his feelings. At other times just the opposite:

Relaxed with Paul: comfortable, contented, cozy, secure; "I could talk to him about anything"; "It's nice to know he's somewhere in the house, even if we're not doing things together right now."

Close to Paul: engaged with, excited by, having a lot to say to, feeling intimate with, looking forward to being with, sexually interested in him. At other times:

Distant from Paul: disconnected from, feeling blah toward, in a rut with, not having much to say to, not feeling intimate with, not looking forward to being with, feeling sexually turned off by him.

Taken for granted by Paul: feeling unnoticed, unappreciated, unimportant to him; "He's married to his work and not to me"; "I'm low on his priority list." At other times:

Not taken for granted by Paul: feeling noticed by him, appreciated by him, important to him.

Taking Paul for granted: not thinking about or appreciating him, involved with the kids or work and not with him, seeing him as someone she has to fit into her schedule. At other times:

Not taking Paul for granted: thinking about him, noticing his moods, rediscovering things to appreciate in him.

Loved by Paul: feeling cared for by, admired by, cherished by, prized by him. At other times:

Hated by Paul: feeling blamed, criticized, disapproved of; feeling that she rubs him the wrong way—that she has lost his good will; "He sees me as the problem," "as a pest," "as the enemy."

Loving Paul—feeling lucky to be married to him: thinking only about his good qualities, struck by what is special about him, appreciating how he takes more responsibility for the house and kids than almost any husband she knows. At other times:

Hating Paul—feeling unlucky to be married to him: thinking only about his bad qualities (having trouble remembering any good ones); noticing that although he does a lot around the house and with the kids, he is only doing a good job of "helping" her, and it is still she who has to make sure that things get done; seeing him as the problem.

Marie generally thinks of herself as having a relationship with Paul. She does not realize that she is having *many* relationships—and such diverse ones. When she rushes into the living room and says, "You never talk to me any more," she has shifted from a person who feels okay about her husband to a person who wants revenge:

Marie suddenly remembers all the wrongs that Paul has ever done her.

Marie suddenly forgets all the other more positive relationships she has with Paul. She cannot remember what it is like to feel glad to be married to him.

She has shifted into the "blaming-Paul, hating-Paul" state of mind. But how has this happened? It requires several steps:

Marie started down the hall in the "self-sympathetic, the-sensitive-way-I-responded-to-Billy-shows-I'm-a-good-mother-and-that, therefore, I-deserve-things, and-I-know-what-I-want: Paul's-attention" state of mind.

But immediately Marie felt, "It's childish and dependent for me to want Paul to listen every time I have a little problem." She snapped into the "self-blame" state of mind.

Which she dealt with by shifting again into the "justifying" state of mind: "It's a husband's duty to listen to his wife when she's had a bad day—especially when she's a working mother struggling under an impossible load."

And, anticipating that Paul wouldn't listen, Marie now finds herself justifying the resentment she felt. She sees Paul as *shirking* his responsibilities. Whereas a moment ago she saw herself as weak and irresponsible for needing Paul's support, she now sees *him* as irresponsible for not having already offered it.

Suddenly all Marie is aware of is how selfish Paul is, how he lets her down. Suddenly he seems the source of all her problems. Marie has snapped into the "blaming-Paul, Paul-is-the-enemy" state of mind. And she would have snapped into it sooner and more wholeheartedly if Paul had been more clearly provocative:

> If, for example, he had said when he first came home, "Get away from me. I don't want to hear about your problems now—I'm not in the mood. Just go and make dinner."
>
> Or if he had called out from the living room, "Bring me a beer, will you?"—treating her as a servant.

In the state of mind Marie was in earlier, she wanted Paul to listen to her. In the state of mind she is in now—the "blaming-Paul, hating-Paul" state of mind—she wants to punish him, to exact her pound of flesh, or at least to get him to admit the wrong he has done her. Flipping into a new state of mind means having a new set of feelings and wishes.

There is this whole other Marie—this whole other way of being—that she has snapped into. When she rushes into the living room and says, "You never talk to me any more," Paul is no longer dealing with a wife who seems content to fix his dinner. He is dealing with a wife who wants to fix *him*.

CHAPTER 10

Defensiveness:
A Multiplicity of Defensive Responses

Much of the problem of defensiveness is that it is hard to recognize. So this chapter presents a list of 44 types of defensive responses to help recognize it.

Paul is watching the News when Marie appears at the door and says:

You never talk to me any more.

What does Paul do? What practically everyone does in such a situation: become defensive. Many, many possible defensive responses occur to him, although he doesn't recognize them as such. He sees them simply as stating the truth, pointing out reality, and setting Marie straight. In fact, Paul would be astonished to hear them labeled "defensive," since they just seem to him the logical points to make.

Astonishing also is the *length* of the list—it keeps going. And the fact that it keeps going reveals how creative Paul is (as are we all) in coming up with defensive responses and in organizing counterattacks. Our partners, of course, are equally creative in *countering* our defensive responses and counterattacks.

The Multitude of Defensive Responses That Occur to Paul

Denying

In response to Marie's, "You never talk to me any more," Paul could say:

1. That's not so; what are you talking about?: "I talk to you all the time."

2. Here's evidence: "What about Wednesday, when you were upset about your mother and we spent the whole evening talking about it?"

3. I was just about to do it: "I was just on my way to the kitchen to talk to you."

4. I'm an innocent bystander: "What have I done now? I've been sitting here bothering nobody, relaxing after a hard day, just wanting some peace and quiet. What's the big problem?"

Explaining (Making Excuses)

In response to Marie's "You never talk to me any more," Paul could say:

5. I didn't know you felt that way: "Why didn't you tell me you wanted to talk? I'm not a mind reader."

6. I thought it was what you wanted: "You were with people all day today. I thought you wanted time to yourself."

7. It's normal: "Married people talk a lot less after a few years. They've already said everything."

8. It's a simple misunderstanding: "I thought it was understood that we'd each take a little time for ourselves and *then* we'd talk."

9. We have different styles: "We're just used to different things. Your family talks a lot. In my family they hardly talk at all."

10. I'm just not good at it: "I don't have a knack for small talk. I never did."

11. There are extenuating circumstances: "I know I haven't been very communicative lately, but I've been under a lot of pressure at work."

Counterattacking

The principle underlying the third type of defensive response is that "the best defense is a good offense." In response to Marie's "You never talk to me any more," Paul could say:

12. You do the same thing/You did it first/You do it, not me: "What about last night, when I was upset and wanted to talk and you spent the whole night working on a memo for the office?"

13. What you do is *worse*: "I'd talk to you more often if you weren't such a *nag*."

14. You're inconsistent: "Last Saturday after the party you said I talked too *much*. Make up your mind, will you?"

15. I did it only in reaction to what *you* did: "I'm not going to feel much like talking when you hit me with all the problems of the day before I even get my coat off."

16. You go too far in the opposite direction: "You always have to talk everything into the ground."

17. What you see as a problem in me is actually a problem in you: "I just don't believe in gossiping."

18. I have a right: "I work all day taking care of other people's problems. I have a right to a little peace and quiet when I come home."

19. You should have told me: "How was *I* to know that you wanted to talk?"

20. You should have told me *sooner:* "If that's what's been bothering you, why did you wait so long to tell me about it? I hate the way you always brood about things and let them build up."

21. You should have told me in a nicer way: "Well, you don't have to be so nasty about it."

22. You knew what you were getting, so you have only yourself to blame: "You knew I wasn't much of a talker when you married me."

23. You should try to be more accepting: "You need to learn to accept people the way they are instead of trying to change them."

24. You have unrealistic expectations: "You can't expect just one person to satisfy all your needs."

25. It's your problem, so you should take care of it: "If you feel a need to talk, you should call up one of your friends."

26. You had the problem long before you met me: "You had the same complaint about your last two boyfriends. So the problem is you, not me."

27. You make the same complaint about everyone else; that ought to tell you something: "You say the same thing about your father and your brother."

28. You're immature (weak, inadequate, crazy, dependent): "You want a mother, not a husband."

29. You're a bottomless pit: "Nothing's ever going to satisfy you. Even if I talked more, you'd just find something else to complain about."

30. I'm your whipping boy: "I'm tired of your taking it out on me when it's really your boss (or your father) you're angry at."

31. You're putting up a smokescreen: "You're blaming me so you don't have to look at your own problems."

32. It's a minor infraction, which brings us to the real problem, which is that you always make such a big deal about everything: "I'm tired of your always complaining." Or "Why are you always so judgmental and hypercritical?" Or "Did we get up on the wrong side of the bed again?" Or "You must be getting your period." Or "You're oversensitive." Or "you're overreacting."

33. You've got a negative attitude: "Why can't you appreciate the good things we have instead of always dwelling on the bad? You worry about things too much and let them bother you more than you should."

34. You must enjoy being unhappy: "You're having a wonderful time feeling sorry for yourself, wallowing in self-pity, and crying about how awful everything is."

35. You're trying to control me: "You're always looking for ways to put me down. You're trying to manipulate me. You want me under your thumb."

36. Things have been too good between us lately, so you're trying to ruin them: "I don't think you *want* things to work out between us. I don't believe for a moment that you really think it's a problem. You're looking for an excuse to feel things are bad. Well, I'm not going to play your game."

Self-Accusing

The purpose of the fourth type of response is not necessarily defensive; Paul may simply *feel* self-accusing. The effect, however, is to draw attention away from Marie's concern and to refocus it on himself. In response to Marie's "You never talk to me any more," Paul could say:

37. You're right: "I blew it again. It's my fault. I keep letting you down. Maybe I'm just incapable of having an adult relationship."

Fixing (Rushing Past the Problem to Find a Solution)

In response to Marie's "You never talk to me any more," Paul could say:

38. I'll fix it: "Well, what exactly do you want to talk about?"

39. I've improved: "You must admit that I'm better than I used to be."

40. I'm trying: "I know it might not be apparent to you yet—I change very slowly—but for me, in my own way, I've made a lot of improvement."

41. I can't change, so you'll have to accept it—and *that's* the solution: "I've never been much of a talker. You'll just have to learn to live with it."

Withdrawing

In response to Marie's "You never talk to me any more," Paul could do the following:

42. Try to put her off: "Can't we talk about it later?"

43. Exit psychologically: Paul could shrug, say nothing, and remain detached for the rest of the evening. Later, he might close the door in such a way that Marie would be unable to tell whether or not he was slamming it.

44. Exit physically: "I'm not going to sit here and listen to this; I'm going out for some air."

Paul's Sorting of the Responses

How does Paul choose among these 44 possibilities? With only a vague awareness of what he is doing, he sorts through them.

He sorts the following 18 responses into the "reject-immediately, she'll-be-able-to-answer-it-too-easily, I-know-exactly-what-she-will-say" category:

Paul's Response to Marie's "You Never Talk to Me Any More"	*What Paul Fears Marie Will Answer*
That's not so: "I talk to you all the time." (1)	"Oh, yeah? Like when?"
I was just about to do it: "I was just on my way to the kitchen to talk to you." (3)	"Oh, really? You look pretty settled there to me, what with your feet on the table and your shoes off."
I thought it was what you wanted: "You were with people all day today. I thought you wanted time to yourself." (6)	"That's what *you* wanted. Let's get it straight."
It's normal: "Married people talk a lot less after a few years. They've already said everything." (7)	"You're *super*normal then, because you don't say *anything*."
It's a simple misunderstanding: "I thought it was understood that we'd take a little time for ourselves and *then* we'd talk." (8)	"I don't remember any such understanding. All I remember is your hightailing it for the TV."
There are extenuating circumstances: "I know I haven't been very communicative lately, but I've been under a lot of pressure at work." (11)	"You're *always* under a lot of pressure at work—which is *something else* I want to talk to you about."
You're inconsistent: "Last Saturday after the party you said I talked too	"Yes, now that you bring that up: Why is it that you have so much

much. Make up your mind, will you?" (14)

to say to everyone else and so little to say to me?"

You go too far in the opposite direction: "You always have to talk everything into the ground." (16)

"Whenever I put two sentences together, you think I'm talking things into the ground."

What you see as a problem in me is actually a problem in you: "I just don't believe in gossiping." (17)

"I'm not talking about gossiping. I'm talking about *talking.*"

You should have told me: "How was I to know that you wanted to talk?" (19)

"It's me, you know, Marie; I *always* want to talk."

You should have told me in a nicer way: "Well, you don't have to be so nasty about it." (21)

"When I tell you in a nicer way, you don't listen then, either."

You have unrealistic expectations: "You can't expect just one person to satisfy all your needs." (24)

"Well, maybe I should look for someone who will satisfy at least *some* of them."

You make the same complaint about everyone else; that ought to tell you something: "You say the same thing about your father and your brother." (27)

"Yeah, you're just like them." (Paul thinks: I don't want Marie to include me in *that* company.)

You're immature (weak, inadequate, crazy, dependent): "You want a mother, not a husband." (28)

"Yes, and look what I got: a husband who's like another child."

You're trying to control me: "You're always looking for ways to put me down. You're trying to manipulate me." (35)

"You're trying to manipulate *me* by refusing to talk to me."

I've improved: "You must admit that I'm better than I used to be." (39)

"I hate to tell you this, but I don't see any change."

I can't change, so you'll have to accept it: "I've never been much of a talker. You'll just have to learn to live with it." (41)

"Well you'd *better* change—because I *can't* live with it."

Try to put her off: "Can't we talk about it later?" (42)

"You won't want to talk about it later, either."

Paul sorts the following 12 responses into the "prime-candidates, these-are-really-good, Marie-won't-know-how-to-answer-these, they-ought-to-do-the-trick" column:

Paul's Response	*His Comments*
Here's evidence: "What about Wednesday, when you were upset about your mother and we spent the whole evening talking about it?" (2)	That could prove her wrong, or at least make her stop and think for a minute.
I'm an innocent bystander: "What have I done now? I've been sitting here bothering nobody, relaxing after a hard day, just wanting some peace and quiet. What's the big problem?" (4)	That's perfect—it establishes just the right tone of startled innocence.
I didn't know you felt that way: "Why didn't you tell me you wanted to talk? I'm not a mind reader." (5)	She might buy that. After all, she knows I'm not a mind reader.
We have different styles: "We're just used to different things. Your family talks a lot. In my family they hardly talk at all." (9)	That's what she's always telling *me*—so she'd have to accept it.
I'm just not good at it: "I don't have a knack for small talk." (10)	That's good. I'd be admitting something, but not much. Small talk is "small," after all.
You do the same thing: "What about last night, when I was upset and wanted to talk and you spent the whole night working on a memo for the office?" (12)	That's *really* good. Not only does it demolish Marie's complaint, but it lets me slip in that I don't like her bringing work home.
I did it only in reaction to what *you* **did:** "I'm not going to feel much like talking when you hit me with all the problems of the day before I even get my coat off." (15)	That's good. Powerful, but not permanently damaging.
I have a right: "I spend all day talking to other people. I have a right to a little peace and quiet when I come home." (18)	It would make her feel too selfish to argue with that.
You should have told me *sooner:* "If that's what's been bothering you, why did you wait so long to tell me about it?" (20)	How could *anyone* argue with something that obvious?
You knew what you were getting: "You knew I wasn't much of a talker when you married me." (22)	She has to accept some of the responsibility.

**You should try to be more
accepting**: "You need to learn to
accept people the way they are instead of trying to change them." (23)

I've been wanting to say that for
a long time.

I'll fix it: "Well, what exactly do
you want to talk about?" (38)

That puts the ball back in her
court.

Paul sorts the following nine responses into the "reject-immediately,
it's-*too*-powerful, it-would-upset-Marie-too-much-and-ruin-the-evening,
it's-not-worth-it" category:

Paul's Response	*Paul's Reservation*
What you do is *worse*: "I'd talk to you more often if you weren't such a nag." (13)	That would really hurt Marie. She hates it when I call her a nag.
You had the problem long before you met me: "You had the same complaint about your last two boy-friends. So the problem is you, not me." (26)	Last time I said this, Marie didn't speak to me for the rest of the evening.
You're a bottomless pit: "Nothing's ever going to satisfy you. Even if I talked more, you'd just find some-thing else to complain about." (29)	Last time I said this, Marie didn't talk to me for the rest of the *week*.
I'm your whipping boy: "I'm tired of your taking it out on me when you're really angry at your boss." (30)	Last time I said this, I had to sleep on the couch.
You're putting up a smokescreen: "You're blaming me so you don't have to look at your own prob-lems." (31)	I don't want to start a war.
You always make such a big deal about everything: "You must be getting your period." (32)	I'd have to be crazy.
You've got a negative attitude: "Why can't you appreciate the good things we have instead of always dwelling on the bad? You worry about things too much and let them bother you more than you should." (33)	There's some truth to this, but she'd get mad if I pointed it out.

You must enjoy being unhappy: "You're having a wonderful time feeling sorry for yourself, wallowing in self-pity, and crying about how awful everything is." (34)

That's overkill. Even *I* don't believe it.

Things have been too good between us lately, so you're trying to ruin them: "I don't think you *want* things to work out between us. You're looking for an excuse to feel things are bad. Well, I'm not going to play your game." (36)

Last time I said that, Marie yelled at me for 10 minutes and was depressed for 2 days. I certainly don't want to repeat that.

Paul sorts the following three responses into the "reject, it's-too-passive" category:

Paul's Response

Paul's Reservation

You're right: "I blew it again. I keep letting you down. Maybe I'm just incapable of having an adult relationship." (37)

Wimpy. And it's giving Marie ammunition she can use against me in the future.

I'm trying: "I know it might not be apparent to you yet—I change very slowly—but for me, in my own way, I've made a lot of improvement." (40)

Mealy-mouthed.

Exit psychologically: I could keep quiet and hope she goes away. (43)

That's wimpy too—but I'm tempted. Maybe I could sort of do it with dignity.

Paul sorts the following two responses into the "it's-not-worth-it-because-of-its-negative-side-effects" category:

Paul's Response

Paul's Reservation

It's your problem, so you should take care of it: "If you feel a need to talk, you should call up one of your friends." (25)

Marie already talks to her friends too much. I don't want to encourage that.

Exit physically: "I'm going out for some air." (44)

It's raining.

So that is how Paul sorts through these 44 defensive responses.

Skeptic: Wait a minute. I don't really see why you call them "defensive." To me they're just ordinary things people say to each other all the time.

Wile: A lot of the ordinary things that people say to each other all the time *are* defensive. Or they're accusing, which then gets the *other* person defensive.

Skeptic: But . . .

Wile: Such accusing and defensiveness are so common that we accept them as the norm. We're so used to slipping in and out of fighting while thinking we're just talking that we hardly know we're doing it.

Skeptic: Well, people shouldn't be so thin-skinned that a little fighting gets them down.

Wile: But they don't *realize* they're fighting. They don't realize that they're being accusing or defensive. That's the point of my listing these 44 defensive responses—to help them realize it.

Skeptic: But I *still* don't see why you call these responses defensive. Okay, maybe some of them are—but a lot of them seem right to the point. Maybe Paul *didn't* know that Marie wanted to talk. Maybe she *does* have an unrealistic view of marriage. Maybe she *is* blaming Paul when she's really angry at her boss. And I don't see what is so wrong with Paul saying, "Well, what exactly do you want to talk about?" I say that all the time to my husband. In fact, I say *many* of these things all the time. Why do you have to call them "defensive"?

Wile: Because they are not responsive to what the other person just said. They're attempts to dilute or refute it rather than to listen to it and consider it. They're part of an argument rather than part of a conversation. Paul's "Well, what exactly do you want to talk about?" is a way to avoid what Marie wants to discuss: her discouragement and resentment about their *lack* of talking. By pinning her down to "exactly" what she wants to say, he's trying to sweep her feelings under the rug while appearing to give her what she wants.

Skeptic: I've got to tell you, this whole list makes me nervous. At one time or another, I've said practically everything on it.

Wile: I'm glad to hear that. I was *hoping* to capture what we all do.

Skeptic: I feel you've caught me doing something wrong—something I *shouldn't* be doing.

Wile: Well, I'm *sorry* to hear that—because the point of the list *isn't* to "catch" you being defensive, but to help you recognize when you are. That's the problem: thinking you're *not* fighting, that only your partner is—which leads you to the discouraging conclusion that your partner is just a difficult, irrational person who fights for no reason at all and is just impossible to talk to. This list is intended to show that you are fighting too. Lots of times the fight shifts from the issue that began it to the issue of who started it or escalated it. You accuse your partner of being accusing or defensive, of insisting on continuing this fight even though it's clearly going nowhere, of running away instead of sticking around to try to work things out, or of taking too long to get over the fight. At such times, it's easy to feel that you're not fighting; it's just your partner who is. And if you *don't* know you're fighting, you're just fighting to prove that you're not. That's where the list comes in: It can show you *how* you are fighting. By demonstrating how you are contributing to the fight, this list can rescue you from the nowhere place of thinking that only your partner is fighting.

CHAPTER 11

The Fight

It doesn't take much for partners to snap into an "adversarial-adversarial" state.

Paul has just sorted through the 44 defensive responses outlined in Chapter 10. But which one does he choose? He picks Response 4: **I'm an innocent bystander.** He chooses it because he feels it strikes just the right tone of startled, injured innocence. In answer to Marie's "You never talk to me any more," he says:

> What have I done now? I've been sitting here bothering nobody, relaxing after a hard day, just wanting some peace and quiet. What's the big problem?

Paul thinks that Marie will have a hard time answering this. But she doesn't:

> Don't act so surprised. You know *exactly* what I'm talking about. You never talk to me—not even tonight, when I really needed it.

Paul hurriedly sorts through his list of defensive responses. This time he chooses Response 5: **I didn't know you felt that way.**

> Why didn't you tell me you wanted to talk? I'm not a mind reader.

But that doesn't work either. Marie replies:

> How could you possibly *not* know? I told you how everything went wrong today.

By this time Paul wishes that he had opted for Response 43: saying nothing and waiting for Marie to go away. But it's too late. So Paul grits his teeth and tries to come up with an example to prove Marie wrong; that is, he makes Response 2: **Here's evidence.**

> What about Wednesday, when you were upset about your mother and we spent the whole evening—

Marie interrupts:

> I remember it well. You said, "Oh, that's too bad," and spent the whole evening watching television.

Paul has forgotten that he hadn't really talked to Marie on Wednesday either. He tries to recoup with Response 6: **I thought it was what you wanted.**

> You were with people all day today. I thought you wanted time to yourself.

Marie quickly disposes of that also:

> Did I look tonight as if I wanted to be left alone? I was reaching out.

No matter what Paul says, Marie is going to surprise him. That is because she has her own arsenal of attacking responses to deal with whatever defensive responses he makes. Not knowing what else to do, Paul resorts to Response 24, which he rejected a moment ago because he felt that Marie would dispose of it too easily: **You have unrealistic expectations.**

> You can't expect just one person to satisfy all your needs.

And Marie *does* have an easy time answering it:

> Well, maybe I should look for someone who will satisfy at least *some* of them.

Which is exactly the reply Paul feared she would make. Quickly he counters with Response 33, which he *also* rejected a moment ago, seeing it as too powerful: **You've got a negative attitude.** But, frustrated by his inability to affect Marie—to get her to back off—his fear at the moment is only that what he says might not be powerful enough:

Why can't you appreciate the good things we have instead of always dwelling on the bad? You worry about things too much and let them bother you more than you should.

Marie winces. She fears that Paul is right and that she *does* have a negative attitude. She sorts through her own list of defensive responses and comes up with her own version of Response 1: **That's not so.**

I *don't* dwell on the bad.

That's pretty lame. Paul feels he has her on the run.

You don't? Tonight is a perfect example. First you bellyache that the kids misbehaved, then, hardly missing a beat, you complain that I don't talk enough. You call that dwelling on the *good* things?

Paul thinks he has her now. But at the last moment she deftly turns it back on him:

It's hard to dwell on the good things when you're married to someone who never talks to you.

Which puts Paul back on the defensive. So he sorts through his list of defensive responses and comes up with Response 38—giving Marie what she says she wants:

Well, what exactly do you want to talk about?

But it turns out *not* to be what she wants.

MARIE: That's not the point now.
PAUL: You said you wanted to talk—so here I am, right here, ready to talk. Go ahead.
Marie: You don't get it, do you?

Paul thinks that he is making a serious offer. He has forgotten all the strategizing he has been doing. And he fails to realize that his "Well, what exactly do you want to talk about?" sounds grudging; it is a challenge rather than an offer. He is saying, in essence, "If it's so important, okay, we'll talk. But *you're* the one who wants to talk—I'd rather watch the News. So it's up to you; there is nothing I want to say." Paul is offering no help and, in addition, is implying that what she says had better be worth his while.

Since Paul thinks he is making a serious offer, he is forced to conclude that Marie will not respond to a serious offer. "She's irrational,"
he tells himself; "There's no way to talk to her." And he snaps out
Response 29: **You're a bottomless pit.**

I get it, all right. Nothing's ever going to satisfy you.

Paul is in no mood for an argument—but that is what he gets. Marie
retorts:

Well, it wouldn't take much to satisfy me. Just a little human treatment.

Totally frustrated, Paul lashes out with Response 13, which he has
held back until now in fear it would ruin the evening. But right now it
doesn't matter; as far as he is concerned, the evening is already ruined.

I'd give you a little human treatment if you weren't such a *nag*.

Paul realizes that he has done it now. He feels he has lit the fuse
and he had better get out fast. He makes Response 44:

This is stupid. I'm going out for some air.

At the moment he doesn't *care* that it's raining.

MARIE: You'll get pneumonia.
PAUL: That's better than staying in here and having a coronary.

Paul slams the door behind him. Since he sees himself as just *reacting* to Marie's provocation—that is, not as being provocative himself—he
is careful to slam the door by just the amount that he feels emotionally
slammed by Marie.

How does the situation degenerate so quickly? It takes so little—a
single accusing remark from Marie ("You never talk to me any more")
and a defensive one from Paul ("What's the big problem?")—to snap them
into an adversarial state.

I have said throughout this book that life is a sequence of states of
mind over which we have only limited control. *Couple* life is an interaction between the shifting states of mind (over which they have only
limited control) of *two* people.

Skeptic: Stop. I don't want to hear any more. It reminds me too
much of *my* marriage.

Wile: That's good. I was hoping this book would be something people could relate to.

Skeptic: Well, I'm not going to relate to it much longer, because I'm going to stop reading. What's your point, anyway? What are you trying to show?

Wile: I'm trying to show what we're all up against. I'm trying to show how a fight is like a chess match in which each partner tries to anticipate the other's moves and countermoves. I'm trying to show how the issue immediately becomes who's the good guy and who's the bad guy—who's mean, neglectful, irresponsible, unreasonable, or unworthy and who isn't. I'm trying to show that "checkmate" means convincing the opponent that he or she is the bad guy. I'm trying to show that neither partner can achieve this goal because each can counter the other's moves indefinitely. I'm trying to show that even when the match is over it isn't really over. Paul is outside walking around in the rain. Marie is back in the kitchen trying to stay away from the chocolate chips while trying to figure out what happened. But both are continually replaying the conversation in their minds.

Skeptic: But you're just showing that relationships are impossible.

Wile: Well, I'm trying to show that they're *difficult*—and why.

Skeptic: Big difference. How is that going to help anybody?

Wile: It can be *relieving* to appreciate that relationships are difficult and to realize that *everyone* has trouble with them—because then you won't have to feel there's something uniquely wrong with your relationship, or with you, or with your partner.

Skeptic: That's not relieving—that's depressing. I already know that relationships are difficult. I want to know what to *do* about them. I want answers.

CHAPTER 12

Five Levels of Attack

This chapter provides a means for measuring the virulence of your own or your partner's attack.

Paul is walking in the rain, feeling angry at Marie. He is getting wet—there was no time to grab an umbrella. But he is happy not to be inside. Marie is there—and she is even angrier at him than he is at her. He, after all, did manage to get in the last word.

How might things have gone better?

Should Marie have simply withheld her anger? Well, sure, except that her "You never talk to me any more" just slipped out. Even if she had been able to catch it in time, she would probably have blurted out another accusation later. Few people are able to suppress anger without letting it escape eventually. "Everybody can act nicer than they feel—but only a little nicer and only for a little while," says ego-analytic couples therapist Nan Narboe, elaborating on a statement by the authors of *Liberated Parents/Liberated Children* (1974/1975, p. 137).[1]

Then, should Paul simply have avoided getting defensive? Of course, except that few people are able to remain nondefensive when accused by someone important to them about an issue they are really sensitive about.

Well, then, should Marie have simply not minded *Paul's* getting defensive? Absolutely, except that few people are able to tolerate defensiveness by someone important to them about an issue they really want this person to understand.

A fight, once started, has its own momentum. Each step leads inevitably to the next:

Marie attacked ("You never talk to me any more").
Which got Paul defensive.

[1]The authors, Adele Faber and Elaine Mazlish, attribute the idea to their mentor, child psychologist Haim Ginott.

Which made Marie feel that she wasn't getting her point across.
Which led her to intensify her attack.
Which got Paul more defensive—that is, even *less* able to listen.
Which made Marie feel even more that she wasn't getting her point
   across.
Which led her to increase her attack.
And on and on.

So if Marie is going to attack, and if Paul is going to get defensive, and if the fight is going to have its own momentum, what do I recommend? As surprising as it might seem, I recommend that Marie and Paul become *experts* in observing their attack and defense patterns.

- That is the purpose of the 44 defensive responses—to help people recognize when they or their partners become defensive. I want them to pin up this list on their mental bulletin boards.
- And beside it, I want them to pin the following list of five levels of attack—to help them recognize when they are escalating their attack, or when their partners are.

Many of the responses that I have labeled as "defensive" in Chapter 10, I label as "attacking" here. In fact, almost any attacking response can also be a defensive response. This is consistent with the idea that "the best defense is a good offense."

A Level 1 Attack: Criticizing Behavior

Marie and Paul's fight began with a Level 1 attack. Marie criticized Paul's behavior ("You never talk to me any more"), which Paul defended against by pointing to *other* behavior ("What about Wednesday, when you were upset about your mother and we spent the whole evening talking about it?"), which Marie also criticized ("You said 'Oh, that's too bad' and spent the whole evening watching television").

A Level 2 Attack: Criticizing Feelings

A little later Paul escalated to a Level 2 attack: He criticized Marie's *feelings*. He told her, "You should appreciate the good things we have instead of always dwelling on the bad. You worry about things too much and let them bother you more than you should."

In so saying, Paul was dealing with Marie's telling him what he should and should not *do* by telling her what she should and should not *feel*. People typically get upset when told what they should and should not feel—even more so than when told how to behave. That is because people cannot control what they feel, whereas they can at least to some extent control what they do.

Of course, people *try* to control what they feel. Marie has already tried to stop dwelling on the bad and to stop worrying so much. After all, neither of these things is any fun for her either.

But it is hard for people to talk themselves out of their worries, dissatisfactions, and feelings. The best Marie can do is to try to distract herself, for example, by going to a movie. And even then, the troubling feeling is likely to spring to mind when she stands in line for popcorn.

But why did Paul shift to a Level 2 attack, even though he knew it would just get Marie more upset? He did it because the ease with which Marie countered each of his defensive responses left him feeling frustrated and powerless.

A Level 3 Attack: Criticizing Character—Name Calling

When, a little later, Marie criticized Paul for not giving her "just a little human treatment," that was more than Paul could stand. He felt even more frustrated and powerless, which led him to escalate to Level 3: criticizing Marie's *character*. He told her, "I'd give you a little human treatment if you weren't such a *nag*."

"You're a nag," like "You're a wimp," "You're a baby," "You're a flake," or "You're castrating," is name calling. It's one of those stop-you-in-your-tracks putdowns.

In making a Level 3 attack, Paul was doing what the books on child rearing warn you not to do. You are not supposed to criticize a child as a person—just the child's behavior. In the language of this chapter, these books are saying: Make Level 1 attacks rather than Level 3 attacks. You're not supposed to say, "You're a bad boy, Billy"—but rather, "I don't like your fighting with your sister."

Similarly, Paul is not supposed to tell Marie, "You're irresponsible—but rather, "I don't like it when you come home late." He is not supposed to say, "You're a nag"—but rather, "I don't like it when you criticize me."

And now we see why, despite these books, Paul *does* at times tell Billy, "You're a bad boy"—and why he *does* at times tell Marie, "You're irresponsible" or "You're a nag." He does so because he is momentarily in the "hating-Billy" or "hating-Marie" state of mind. He thinks Billy *is* "a bad boy." He thinks Marie *is* "irresponsible" or "a nag." All his senses tell him so. Paul's state of mind determines his reality, and, at these moments, Paul is in the "Billy-is-defective" or "Marie-is-defective" state of mind.

A Level 4 Attack: Making Accusatory Interpretations

Paul's calling Marie a nag ended the conversation—he felt he had to get out of there. If it had not ended the conversation, however, Marie or Paul might eventually have escalated to a Level 4 attack: making accusatory interpretations. Paul might tell Marie, "I'm tired of your blaming me when you're really angry at your boss." And Marie might answer, "Well, *I'm* tired of your seeing me as your mother hammering at you to do this and not do that."

In the first three levels of attack, Paul was telling Marie that something was wrong with what she *does* (Level 1), what she *feels* (Level 2), and who she *is* (Level 3). In the fourth level of attack, he would be telling her *why* she has this problem. He would be tracing her problem to childhood or describing her defenses or psychological complexes.

Is a Level 4 attack more provocative than the other three? Not necessarily. Calling Marie a "nag," which was a Level 3 attack, was the major blow—the knife thrust to the heart. Marie was sensitive to this charge. Interpreting—that is, telling her *why* she is a nag ("blaming me when you're really angry at your boss")—would simply twist the knife by adding another increment of provocation.

People do not like being told that they are taking out on people the anger they have toward someone else in their lives. They feel invaded. They think their minds are being played with. They feel they are being "psychoanalyzed." And they worry that the attacker may be right.

A Level 5 Attack: Criticizing Intentions

If he felt sufficiently frustrated and powerless, Paul might escalate to the fifth level—interpreting Marie's *intentions*:

> I don't believe it for a minute. You're making up these problems in order to make me feel guilty. You're trying to punish me. Things have been too good between us lately, and you're trying to ruin them. I think you want to be unhappy. I don't think you want things to work out between us. You're trying to destroy the relationship.

Marie would be stunned. Paul's charges would seem to her so off the wall—so far from anything she was feeling—that she would hardly know how to begin to answer them:

What are you talking about?

In his present state of mind, Paul would take this as pretended innocence:

You know *exactly* what I'm talking about. You set the whole thing up. You *wanted* us to fight. You're sitting there gloating, loving every minute of it.

And now Marie would be *really* bewildered:

That's ridiculous. I'm *hating* every minute of it. Not only am I not gloating, I hate fighting so much I feel physically ill. And I certainly didn't set it up. If I had, I sure would have made it work out better.

This would be a powerful rebuttal. Paul, however, might be undeterred:

I didn't say you did it deliberately. You set the whole thing up *unconsciously.*

Marie would be speechless. There would be no way for her to refute this charge. In her frustration, all she might be able to do would be to throw a tantrum—or withdraw and feel totally helpless.

Paul would be seeing Marie as an all-powerful, totally-in-charge malevolent force. In his view, whatever happened would be what Marie wanted to happen. If they had a fight, she must have wanted them to fight. If she suffered, she must have wanted to suffer. If she set him up in a way that did not work out well for her, she must have had her reasons for that, too.

It is clear why a Level 5 attack is more provocative than the other four. Paul would have gone beyond criticizing Marie's actions (Level 1), feelings (Level 2), and character (Level 3)—and beyond making psychodynamic interpretations (Level 4). He would be shaking her sense of reality (Level 5). In making a Level 2 attack, he was telling Marie what she *should* want; in making a Level 5 attack, he would be telling her what she *does* want—and that there is something very wrong with her for wanting it.

This would be the "hating-my-partner, feeling-done-in-by-my-partner-and-lashing-back" state of mind in full flower. Paul would see Marie as having malicious intent ("You're trying to punish me"), as manipulating him ("You set the whole thing up"). He would see her as *wanting* to produce the negative effect she was having on him ("You're trying to make me feel guilty") as well as on herself ("I think you want to be unhappy") and on them both as a couple ("You're trying to destroy the relationship"). And he would see her as getting secret enjoyment from what she is doing ("You're loving every minute of it").

Paul would be *convinced* that Marie was doing (or getting) these things. Our state of mind determines our reality, and, at the moment, Paul would be in the "hating-Marie, Marie-is-trying-to-do-me-in-and-possibly-also-trying-to-do-herself-in" state of mind.

And that is what I would believe too if I were Paul and were in the Level 5, "hating-Marie" state of mind. I would have no choice, just as Paul would have no choice.

Being Aware of the Levels

And that is where I want Paul and Marie to start: with the recognition that when they are at any given level, they have no choice but to be at that level.

I want them to *know* the level they are at:

If Paul says to Marie, "You're always criticizing me," I want him to know that he is at Level 1. He is criticizing Marie's behavior—and she is going to be upset.

And if Paul says, "And that's because you're overreacting, you're oversensitive, and you worry about things too much," I want Paul to know that he is now at Level 2. He is telling Marie that her feelings are wrong—and she is going to be even more upset.

And if Paul says, "And that's because you're neurotic," I want him to know that he is now at Level 3—he is criticizing her character. And Marie is going to be more upset yet.

And if Paul says, "And that's because you've never dealt with your feelings about your mother," I want him to know that he is now at Level 4. He is telling Marie the origins of her problems. And he should not be surprised if Marie really hits the ceiling.

And if Paul says, "And you're manufacturing complaints so you can blame the relationship and avoid confronting your own problems," I want him to know that he is now at Level 5. He is telling Marie what her purpose is. And so he should not be surprised if she becomes totally enraged—or totally bewildered.

I want each partner to know that each succeeding level of attack represents a further degree of rage, frustration, and powerlessness on his or her part and is likely to produce a further degree of rage, frustration, and powerlessness on the other partner's part.

I also want Paul to be able to recognize *Marie's* level of attack:

If Marie says, "You never talk to me any more," I want Paul to know that *he* is facing a Level 1 ("something-is-wrong-with-your-behavior") attack. Although it is the mildest level of attack, it can seem provocative enough if he is sensitive to the charge.

And if Marie says, "And that's because you don't have the feelings that a husband should have toward his wife," I want Paul to know that he is now facing a Level 2 ("something-is-wrong-with-your-feelings") attack. Unless he happens to be in a "wonderful, nothing-can-bother-me" state of mind, he is going to feel really provoked.

And if Marie says, "And that's because you're selfish, afraid of comitment, incapable of love, and care only about yourself," I want him to know that he is now facing a Level 3 ("something-is-wrong-with-your-character") attack. Marie has temporarily joined forces with his harsh internal schoolmaster—a lethal combination.

And if Marie says, "And that's because you haven't gotten over your mother's emotionally suffocating you," I want Paul to know that he is now facing a Level 4 ("something -is-wrong-with-your-childhood") attack. I want Paul to understand why he suddenly sees Marie as a self-righteous know-it-all, and, at the same time, begins to worry secretly that she may be right.

And if Marie says, "You're unconsciously trying to destroy the relationship," I want Paul to know that he is now facing a Level 5 ("let-me-tell-you-what-your-unconscious-intentions-are") attack. I want Paul to understand why he suddenly feels totally enraged, bewildered, or trapped and needs to run.

Each succeeding statement represents a further degree of frustration on Marie's part in her effort to get Paul to appreciate how she feels— even though, since each statement is more provocative than the one before, it just further stiffens his resistance.

And what *are* the feelings that Marie wants Paul to appreciate? Her hurt, loneliness, rejection, abandonment, and resentment. (These are the

"I statements" behind Marie's "you statements.") When she says "You're selfish, afraid of commitment, incapable of love, and care only about yourself," she is telling him in essence that she feels unnoticed, insecure, unloved, and lonely. These feelings seem so self-evident to her—so much the dominant thing going on—that the particular words she chooses to describe them seem to her irrelevant.

> She assumes that Paul *has* to know she has these feelings, since they seem so all-consuming to her. She doesn't realize that she hasn't told him that she is having them.
>
> She hasn't told him because she feels *unentitled* to them, despite their being all-consuming. She thinks she is being weak and childish to feel so easily abandoned, lonely, rejected, and unlovable.
>
> So she buttresses her position by accusing Paul of *being* abandoning, neglectful, rejecting, and unloving—in which case, her feelings would be understandable responses. She makes accusations ("you statements") instead of stating feelings ("I statements"). And now we see a major reason for making "you statements" (e.g., "You're unloving") rather than "I statements" (e.g., "I feel unlovable"): It allows people to justify feelings to which they feel unentitled.
>
> She doesn't realize that her harsh, righteous, punitive, scolding tone leaves Paul feeling beaten up rather than informed.
>
> And even if she were to acknowledge it, she would say she is simply being emphatic because he would not listen otherwise.

So, Marie is verbally beating Paul up when she thinks that she is just telling him how she feels. And, in response, he is verbally beating her up when he thinks that he is just setting her straight.

That is what an escalating couple fight is: a self-perpetuating exchange in which two people become increasingly unhearing and abusive because each feels increasingly unheard and abused by the other.

Skeptic: You're obviously having a wonderful time describing how impossible relationships are, while I'm sitting here seeing myself in all your examples, and getting more and more depressed. And again, you keep telling me about the problem, when what I want to hear about is the solution.

Wile: But hearing about the problem *is* the solution. I've been giving the solution all along. Imagine how it would go for Paul and Marie if they had all the information about their fight I've just discussed. Let's imagine that they knew all this:

Marie was attacking, and as a result, Paul was understandably getting defensive.

Paul was getting defensive, and as a result, Marie was understandably getting more provoked.

Each was trying to prove the other wrong and trying to counter the other's effort to do so.

The situation was unresolvable because Paul could always find a defensive response among the 44 potential responses, and Marie could always find a further accusation.

As weapons of attack, they each selected something that they thought the other could not respond to and that would be powerful enough to make an impression, but not powerful enough to really hurt the other. Unless, of course, they each felt so frustrated and powerless that, for the moment, they didn't care if they *did* hurt the other.

There were five successive levels of attack to which Paul or Marie might shift as they felt increasingly threatened, frustrated, and powerless.

Skeptic: That's all very nice, but how would knowing all this really help?

Wile: Think about it. If Marie and Paul were to know all these things—let's say they had read these chapters—then they couldn't have had the fight in quite the same way:

If Marie had known that her "You never talk to me any more" was an attack—and not, as she thought, simply an expression of her feelings—then she wouldn't have had to conclude that Paul got defensive without reason and there wasn't a way to talk to him.

If Paul had known that he wasn't trying to reason with Marie (which is what he thought he was doing), but instead was spewing out one defensive response after another—that is, if he had tacked up the list of 44 defensive responses on his mental bulletin board and could recognize when he was using them—he'd be able to understand why Marie wasn't listening to him and why things were spiraling out of control. He wouldn't have felt so confused and powerless, and he might never have escalated to a Level 2 attack—telling her she shouldn't be having the feelings she was having. But even if he did, at least he'd know he was doing it— and he wouldn't be so surprised when, in response, Marie just got more upset.

If Paul had known when he said, "Well, what do you want to talk about?" he wasn't giving Marie what she wanted, but instead was being defensive, he wouldn't have had to take Marie's negative reaction as meaning that she was irrational and that there was no way to talk to her.

That is what I'm trying to do in this book: give people a whole new set of ideas that will allow them to lead their lives in a whole new way.

PART 4

IMPLICATIONS FOR COUPLES THERAPY: DEALING WITH ADVERSARIAL STATES

In Chapters 13 and 14, I talk about the adversarial state that exists between partners. In Chapters 15 and 16, I talk about the adversarial state that exists between the therapist and the partners.

CHAPTER 13

What Fighting Is

Everyone knows that fighting—accusation and defensiveness—can be injurious to couple relationships and an impediment to couples therapy. In fact, fighting can be such an impediment to couples therapy (despite whatever unconscious purpose it might be thought to serve) that some therapists are quick to interrupt it. They tell the partners, in one way or another, *not* to accuse and *not* to be defensive.

Yet fighting can offer a clue to important things going on in the relationship. When a client weeps, we know that he or she has hit upon something important; the tears are a clue. The same is true with fighting. When partners fight, we know that they have struck a nerve.

When I do couples therapy, I do what every therapist does: I try to keep order; that is, I try to keep the fight from destroying the therapy. But I also do something else: I try to *use* the partners' fighting as a clue that they have just run into something important.

As soon as I turned my attention from simply trying to eliminate or reduce fighting to using fighting as a clue, I discovered that:

1. People are not good at fighting.
2. They do not *know* that they are fighting.
3. They do not *want* to know.
4. Even if they were to know, they would not want to *admit* it.
5. They think that it is *bad* to fight.

In this chapter, I discuss these five ideas. In the next chapter, I show how these ideas lead to a therapeutic approach based, in part, on improving clients' ability to present their cases.

To demonstrate these five ideas, I present a couples therapy vignette. In Part 2 of this book, I have described a set of individual therapy sessions in which Marie is the client. But for the present purpose let us say that I am seeing both Marie and Paul in couples therapy. The morning after the fight, they come in for their weekly therapy session. It is our fourth meeting.

Early that morning, while taking her shower, Marie puzzles over what happened the night before. She is still smarting over Paul's calling her a nag, but she feels partly to blame. She says to herself:

> Instead of accusing Paul—telling him, "You never talk to me any more"—I should have said, "*We* never talk any more." And instead of blaming him for the problem, I should have attributed it to our busy lives, which is a lot of the problem anyway.

When Marie and Paul come into my office and sit down, Marie turns to Paul and says:

> There's something I wanted to tell you last night, but I didn't do a very good job of it. It's that we hardly get a chance to talk any more. I've gotten so caught up in my job, and in dealing with the kids, and worrying about the kids, and just *being* with the kids—not to mention everything else I have to do—sometimes I even forget that I have a husband.

Paul is glad that Marie seems to have gotten over his hit-and-run "You're a nag" and that she no longer seems angry at him. So he says:

> Well, I'd remind you—except I forget that you have a husband, too. Lately my job alone seems to use up 48 hours a day.

But having re-established a good feeling between them, Marie suddenly becomes aware of her unresolved *bad* feeling. What she was planning to say at this point was "You know, maybe if we helped each other out more with some of our chores, we could clear some time for each other." But what comes out of her mouth instead is this:

> You know, it *would* help if you'd bathe Jeannie once in a while.

Why does Marie so quickly snap out of the "feeling-good-toward-Paul" state of mind and back into the "feeling-bad-toward-Paul" state? When people are in the "feeling-good" state, they lose their ability to complain. They feel they are supposed to be friendly, agreeable, accepting, and tolerant. They switch into what I call the "yes mentality." They feel they are supposed to be good sports, be uncritical, avoid conflict, have a positive attitude, give their partners the benefit of the doubt, and accept their partners the way they are rather than try to change them.

When Marie snaps into the "feeling-good-about-Paul" state and feels she is supposed to accept Paul the way he is, she suddenly has a nightmare vision of the relationship going on as it is now into infinity, with no possibility of change. And she can't stand it. She needs him to change—and she feels she has no way to change him except by complaining. She snaps out of the "feeling-good-about-Paul, yes-mentality, being-friendly, accepting-and-uncomplaining" state and into the "feeling-not-so-good-about-Paul, regaining-my-ability-to-complain" state.

And she blurts out, "You know, it would help if you'd bathe Jeannie once in a while." Paul replies:

That's not fair. I bathed her just last week.

This frustrates Marie because:

Paul's bathing Jeannie *one* time is not the point. Marie wants him to bathe her *regularly* and to remember to do it all by himself.
His bathing Jeannie regularly and not relying on her to remind him is not the point, either—even though Marie herself has brought it up. It is just an *example* of the point, which is that Marie would like him to take equal initiative in doing household chores and taking care of the kids.
Getting him to take equal initiative is not the point, either. Or rather, it is just a secondary point—although an important one. The primary point is that Marie wants more of a sense that she and Paul are in it together.
Furthermore, Paul *didn't* bathe Jeannie last week, as she recalls. It was *2* weeks ago. And he didn't do it to be helpful. He just did it to free up Marie's time so she could type up a roster that he needed for work.
Besides, Marie is still upset about being called a nag.

Marie is unable to tell Paul about any of this. Since she is saying just a sliver of what she really needs to say, she is enraged that he has the nerve to argue with even that.

So what does Marie do in the face of all of this? How does she deal with all the frustrations that are welling up? She replies to Paul's "I bathed her just last week" by saying:

No, you didn't.

To which Paul responds:

Yes, I did.

This exchange brings us to a fact about accusing and defensiveness that everyone knows: It can immediately bring an end to useful discussion and snap the partners into an "adversarial–adversarial" couple state. The almost instinctive reaction that couples therapists have when partners get into such an unproductive argument is to try to think of a way to get them to stop.

> That is much of the idea behind communication skills training: to get partners to communicate in nondefensive and nonattacking ways.
>
> That is one of the reasons why some couples therapists trace problems to childhood. By pointing out that Marie's anger at Paul is really anger at her father, the therapist hopes to defuse the situation.
>
> That is much of the idea behind the strategic therapy approach of prescribing the symptom by telling fighting partners to go home and fight—so that they will go home and *not* fight, or at least so that they will fight in a way that comes more under the control of the therapist.
>
> And that is much of the idea behind creating a platform (my approach). I want to give partners a taste of what it would be like if they were not attacking and if they were not being defensive.

It is understandable that couples therapists devote such effort to getting partners to stop fighting. Couples therapy became feasible only when therapists discovered ways to interrupt the accusations and defensiveness in which partners typically engage when seen together. Before then, many therapists who experimented with conjoint couples therapy became fatalistic when the partners started to fight, concluded that couples therapy was unworkable, and recommended that one or both partners go into long-term individual psychotherapy.

Accusation and defensiveness remain the biggest practical problems of couples therapy today. Therapy with both partners is essentially an experiment to see whether, in this setting, the partners will be able to talk in a less accusing and a less defensive way than they do at home (or, if they don't talk at home, whether in this setting they will be *able* to talk). In some cases, the experiment fails. The partners get into the same kind of slashing, unmanageable fights in the office that they do at home.

A crucial task of couples therapy is to try to keep the fighting from destroying the therapy. But in focusing our attention on reducing fighting, we can easily fail to notice the following important facts about it.

The First Fact of Fighting: Being Inept Fighters

We may fail to notice, first of all, that the accuser is typically doing a poor job of presenting his or her case and the defender is doing a poor job of defending.

Marie responds to Paul's "I bathed her just last week" by saying, "No, you didn't." She thus picks one of the weakest and least satisfying of all the arguments she could make.

Here is what Marie might say, instead of "No, you didn't," if she were really to lay things out:

> I can't stand your arguing with me about whether you bathed Jeannie last week—because even if you did, that's not the point. The point is that you don't bathe her *regularly*. The point is that I'm the one who has to organize everything and make sure it gets done. I thought we had a partnership, but lately I've lost the sense of our being in it together. Something happened to us, something changed, and I'm pretty upset about it.

Now *that* really lays it out. Marie would certainly get a lot of satisfaction out of saying that (while, at the same time, providing Paul a fuller glimpse into her feelings). And, as the therapist, it is my job to help her say it.

And immediately we see the value of therapists' being able to *think* about accusation and defensiveness rather than just trying to stop it. The result is the discovery of a new therapeutic task:

- The old task was to get Marie to stop accusing.
- The new task is to improve her ability to present her case.

But why is Marie unable to say what I have just said for her? Because when people snap into the "accusing" state of mind, they become grim and narrowed-down. They lose the big picture. All they can think of is the last thing the other person said—the last defensive or accusatory statement that was thrown at them. They lose the ability to think, or even remember crucial things they know. Marie cannot say, "I've lost the sense of our being in it together," because in the state of mind she is in, her horizon isn't wide enough for her to pin down that feeling. The "accusing" state of mind is typically a poor one from which to state your case.

There are exceptions, of course. Some people become articulate and energized when switching into the "accusing" state of mind. They remember the big picture; they become better able to think. For them—and perhaps for most of us, at some moments and about some issues—the "accusing" state of mind is a good one from which to state their case. But Marie and Paul are not the exceptions.

While Marie is doing a poor job making her case, Paul is doing a poor job of defending himself. As you remember, he responds to her "No, you didn't" by saying, "Yes, I did." Now, that is not much of a defense; Paul is unlikely to get much satisfaction out of it.

Here is what Paul might say if he were to make a really good—a really satisfying—defense:

> Hey, I thought we were talking about forgetting that we were mar-
> ried—and about how we've drifted apart. But I'm getting the idea
> now that what you really want to do is criticize me for not bath-
> ing Jeannie. Well, okay—if that's what you want to do, criticize
> away. But wake me up when you want to talk about forgetting
> that we're married—because you were really onto something there,
> and that's what *I* want to talk about.

Now *that* is a defense Paul would enjoy.

But why is Paul unable to say such a thing in the first place? Because when people snap into the "defensive" state of mind, they lose much of their ability to defend their case, just as when they are in the "accus-ing" state, they lose much of their ability to prosecute it. Paul cannot say, "Hey, I thought we were talking about forgetting that we were mar-ried," because he cannot remember it—even though he and Marie were talking about it just a moment before. That is what snapping into the defensive state of mind typically does: It makes you forget much of what you know—even if you knew it just seconds ago.

Here again we see the value of therapists' studying couple fighting rather than simply stopping it. The result is the discovery of a new thera-peutic task:

- The old task was to stop Paul from being defensive.
- The new task is to improve his ability to defend—that is, to enable him to launch a more elegant and a more satisfying defense.

When people really want to impress someone, they often find them-selves least able to. They lose all their charm and become bumbling.

Similarly, when people really want to make their case or defend themselves, they often lose their ability to do so.

The Second Fact of Fighting: Not Knowing You Are Fighting

Marie responds to Paul's defensive insistence that he *did* bathe Jeannie last week by becoming more stridently accusing:

You're a liar.

Which leads to Paul's becoming more resolutely defensive:

PAUL: Who are you calling a liar?
MARIE: If the shoe fits . . .
PAUL: Well, the shoe *doesn't* fit.

We now arrive at another fact we would notice if we were to think about fighting: The accuser typically does not know that he or she is being accusing, and the defender typically doesn't know that he or she is being defensive—despite the fact that to everyone else these facts are absolutely clear.

Marie doesn't think she is accusing Paul. She thinks she is just saying what is true: As she recalls, Paul did not bathe Jeannie last week, and so he is a liar for saying he did. She doesn't know that she is in a "narrowed-down, shooting-my-quills, unable-to-think, losing-the-big-picture, unable-to-remember-very-much" state.

Paul does not think he is being defensive. He thinks he is stating plain facts: As he recalls, he *did* bathe Jeannie last week, and so he is *not* a liar. He sees himself as simply "reacting" to Marie's provocation. He does not realize that he is reacting in a "provocative, narrowed-down, pulling-my-shell-around-me, unable-to-think, losing-the-big-picture, losing-my-sense-of-humor, instinctively-refuting-everything-that-Marie-says" way.

It is too bad that Marie does not know that she is being accusing. If she did know, she wouldn't have to conclude (as she does) that Paul gets defensive for no reason at all, and that there is no way to talk to him. She would realize that he is defensive because she is attacking.

And it is too bad that Paul doesn't know that he is being defensive. If he did know, he would not have to conclude that Marie gets angry at him for no reason at all, and that there is no way to talk to her. He would realize that her accusing is, in part, a response to his defensiveness.

The Third Fact of Fighting: Not Wanting to Know That You Are Fighting

Of course, part of the reason why Marie and Paul do not know they are fighting is that they do not want to know. Part of fighting is convincing yourself that you are not fighting; it's just the other person who is— or at least it's the other person who started the fight, escalated it, insisted on continuing the fight even though it was obviously going nowhere, or took too long to get over it.

Thus, when Marie replies to Paul's "Well, the shoe *doesn't* fit" by saying—

Why do you always have to be so defensive?

—Paul tries to convince himself that he is not being defensive (i.e., that he is *not* fighting). He tells himself:

What is Marie talking about? I'm not always defensive. I'm hardly ever defensive. And I'm not being defensive *now*. And if I am, it's only because Marie is attacking me.

So he tells Marie:

Why do you always have to be so critical?

To which Marie responds by telling herself:

What is Paul talking about? I'm not always critical. I'm hardly ever critical, and I'm certainly not being critical *now*.

And she tells Paul:

I'm not being critical; I'm just telling you how I feel.

The Fourth Fact of Fighting: Not Wanting to Admit That You Are Fighting

Why are Marie and Paul trying to convince themselves that they are not fighting? Because, to further develop the point I just made,

Part of accusing is defending yourself against the charge of being accusing, and accusing the other person of being defensive.

Part of being defensive is defending yourself against the charge of being defensive, and accusing the other person of accusing.

Paul has to be prepared at any moment for Marie to say, as she has just done, "Why do you always have to be so defensive?" And he *is* prepared. He immediately shoots back, "Why do you always have to be so critical?"

And he also could say, "Why do you *think*? Listen to your tone of voice."
Or he could simply shrug wearily and say nothing.

Marie has to be prepared, at any moment, for Paul to say, as he has just done, "Why do you always have to be so critical?" And she *is*. She shoots back, "I'm not critical; I'm just telling you how I feel."

And she also could say, "You're oversensitive."
Or "It doesn't matter whether I'm being critical or not; you don't listen to me either way."

Why is it so important for Marie and Paul to convince themselves—and each other—that they are not being accusing or defensive? Because they think they *shouldn't* be these things.

The Fifth Fact of Fighting: Thinking You Should Not Be Fighting

Of course Marie and Paul think they shouldn't be these things. That is what we all think.

We have arrived at the heart of the problem, which is that couples have the same attitude toward fighting that therapists have. Therapists think that it is maladaptive for partners to become accusing and defensive, and they try to stop them from doing so. Partners think that it is maladaptive to become accusing and defensive, and they insist that they are not.

There is an irony here. Marie and Paul's belief that they should not be fighting is largely responsible for their being so poor at presenting their cases. It is hard to develop skill at something you disapprove of and are trying to convince yourself you *aren't* doing. Marie and Paul's belief that they shouldn't be accusing or defensive results in their pursuing inept means of developing their positions. That is, it leads to the "narrowed-down, humorless, losing-the-big-picture, dogged, grabbingby-the-pants-leg, losing-all-sense-of-proportion, denying-that-I-am-being-accusing-or-defensive, provocative" forms of presenting their cases that I have described earlier.

There is a vicious cycle here:

> Marie and Paul's belief that accusation and defensiveness are "bad" leads them to engage in unsatisfying and inept forms of presenting their cases.
> Their unsatisfying and inept forms of presenting their cases reaffirm their belief that accusation and defensiveness are "bad" and that they shouldn't engage in them.

Implications of These Five Typically Unrecognized Problems of Accusation and Defensiveness

To summarize, people are (1) not good at fighting, (2) do not know that they are fighting, (3) do not want to know it, and (4) do not want to admit it, largely because they (5) think they shouldn't be fighting.

But how does our knowing all this help?

> To the degree that partners appreciate that they are not good at fighting—that is, to the degree that they realize that when they fight, they become narrowed down, lose the ability to think, respond simply to the last comment the other person made, and lose the big picture—they will be in a good position, after the fight, to try to puzzle out what their point really *is*.
> To the degree that *therapists* appreciate that partners are not good at fighting, they will be able to devote their therapeutic efforts, not to stopping such fighting, but to improving partners' ability to fight—that is, to helping them make their points in clearer, more satisfying ways.

CHAPTER 14

Dealing with Couple Fighting by Helping Partners Make Their Points

Fighting is a fallback position. It is what people do, among other things, when they are unable to make their points. It is a position that they go to quickly and frequently; people are in an accusing or a defensive state much of the time.

What keeps a fight going—what makes it unresolvable—is this fact that neither partner is able to make any of his or her points. An important part of the therapeutic task, accordingly, is to help them do so and, in the process, do the following things:

1. Tap the fight for what it reveals about the relationship.
2. Improve the partners' ability to fight. People are generally not good at presenting their cases and defending themselves, so I try to improve their ability to do so.
3. Engage the partners *about* their fight, instead of focusing entirely on trying to stop the fight (on the one hand) or simply letting it go on (on the other).

The Couples Session with Marie and Paul

To show how I try to do these things, let us return to this session with Marie and Paul. As you remember from Chapter 13, they begin by saying:

MARIE: There's something I wanted to tell you last night, but I didn't do a very good job of it. It's that we hardly get a chance to talk any more. I've gotten so caught up in my job, and in dealing with the kids, and worrying about the kids, and just *being* with the kids—not to mention everything else I have to do—sometimes I even forget that I have a husband.

PAUL: Well, I'd remind you—except I forget that you have a husband, too. Lately my job alone seems to use up 48 hours a day.

THERAPIST (*to himself*): This has the makings of a great conversation. I'll just sit back and enjoy it.

MARIE (*to Paul*): You know, it *would* help if you'd bathe Jeannie once in a while.

PAUL: That's not fair. I bathed her just last week.

MARIE: No, you didn't.

PAUL: Yes, I did.

THERAPIST (*to himself*): The "great conversation" is degenerating pretty fast. I'd better do something.

MARIE (*to Paul*): You're a liar.

THERAPIST (*to himself*): Too late. Missed my chance. In calling Paul a liar, Marie escalated from a Level 1 attack (criticizing his behavior) to a Level 3 attack (criticizing his character). Let's see if I can find a way to talk with them about it.

THERAPIST (to partners): A moment ago you were having this great conversation and—

PAUL (*to Marie*): Who are you calling a liar?

THERAPIST: A moment ago you were—

MARIE (*to Paul*): If the shoe fits . . .

THERAPIST: A moment—

PAUL (*to Marie*): Well, the shoe *doesn't* fit.

THERAPIST (*to himself*): Oh, so it's going to be one of *those* hours—with Marie and Paul so caught up in their fight they can't hear anything I say. I know what one of my old supervisors, Stevens, would say:

> Don't let Marie and Paul intimidate you, Wile. Assert your authority. *Insist* on being heard. Shout them down if you have to. Tell them, "Wait a minute; I've got something to say" or "Hold on there; we need some ground rules." It's your job to keep things from getting out of control—that's what Marie and Paul are paying you for.

THERAPIST (*to himself*): But another supervisor, Cotton, would say:

> Don't overreact, Wile. So what if they raise their voices? So what if they ignore you and drown you out? The purpose of therapy isn't

to demonstrate your authority. If things get a little heated, be patient, wait for a letup, and then ask them how they feel about the fight. Your job is *not* to panic—that's what Marie and Paul are paying you for.

THERAPIST (*to himself*): And I know what Eccles, yet another voice from the past, would say:

Don't fight them, Wilc. Take whatever they say at the moment and *engage* with them in it. If Marie calls Paul a liar, engage her on that. And engage Paul on how he feels being called a liar. If 2 seconds later they start talking about something else, engage them on the *new* subject. That's how you get their attention and establish order—not by shouting them down and by forcing *them* to stick to the topic, but by sticking with them every time they change the topic. Your job is to meet them where they are at the moment and to develop what they say, not challenge it. That's what Marie and Paul are paying you for.

THERAPIST (*to himself*): And I know what my mentor, Casterhazen, would tell me:

Neither Marie nor Paul can hear what the other says—or what you say—because they're both feeling too unlistened to themselves. They're unable to make their points. Your job is to find a way to help them make their points—that's what Marie and Paul are paying you for.

As Marie and Paul continue to argue, I look for a letup in the fight, as Cotton would do. I try to think of how to engage with them in what they are talking about, as Eccles would advise. I try to think of how to help them make their points, *à la* Casterhazen. And, all the time, I am wondering whether I should do as Stevens would do: insist on being heard and shout them down.

MARIE: Why do you always have to be so defensive?
PAUL: Why do you always have to be so critical?
MARIE: I'm not critical; I'm just telling you how I feel.
PAUL: You're not telling me how you feel; you're criticizing me.

THERAPIST (*to himself*): There's no letup yet.

MARIE: I'm not criticizing; you're oversensitive.
PAUL: You think calling me names isn't criticizing?

THERAPIST (*to himself*): This is getting worse.

MARIE: I didn't call you names.

PAUL: You called me a liar.

MARIE: Well, you called me a nag.

THERAPIST (*to himself*): Maybe there isn't going to be a letup and they're going to fight like this for the rest of the session. Maybe Stevens is right and I should shout them down.

PAUL: But that was yesterday—ancient history. Can't you stick to the subject?

MARIE: That *is* the subject. Why do you think I called you a liar just now? I'm still smarting over your calling me a nag yesterday.

THERAPIST (*to himself*): Now *that* is interesting. If that really *is* why Marie called Paul a liar—and not just something she threw in just as a counterpunch at the moment—then it's something useful to work with. Things are looking up.

PAUL: Well, you should have gotten over it by now.

THERAPIST (*to himself*): *Paul* doesn't think that things are looking up. In fact, he has escalated to a Level 2 attack—telling Marie that she shouldn't feel the way she feels.

PAUL: You should do what I do: get it out and then forget about it.

THERAPIST (*to himself*): I hate it when people tell each other what they should or shouldn't do and feel. I'd like to defend Marie, but I can't think of how to do it without accusing Paul. So I'll just have to let Marie defend herself the best she can.

MARIE: Oh, pooh!

THERAPIST (*to himself*): Well, that's *one* way.

PAUL: Don't "Oh, pooh" me.

In the next 2 seconds, I have the following conversation with myself. Every therapist has such barely conscious internal conversations. A purpose of this book is to draw attention to them, slow them down, turn up the volume, and describe in complete sentences what we typically experience as a set of rapid-fire condensed signals.

My Inner Conversation

There's a letup here, so I could ask Marie and Paul how they feel about the fight—as Cotton would recommend.

Or I could say, "Let's go back to the beginning of the hour. You were having this great conversation in which, Marie, you said that you forgot that you had a husband and then, Paul, you said that you forgot that you *were* a husband. Then all that got lost. What do you think happened?"

Or I could include them in the decision of what to talk about. I could say, "There are several issues on the table—the 'forgetting-about-Paul-being-a-husband' issue, the 'bathing-Jeannie' issue, and the 'liar-and-nag' issue. Which of these should we go into? Or is the fight you're having the crucial issue—and *that's* what we should go into first? Or is there something else entirely, something you haven't mentioned yet, that we should start with?"

What I really want to do is, as Eccles recommends, try to engage with them in what they are talking about. And I want to do it in a way that helps them make their points, as Casterhazen suggests. I'll restate what each just said, but in a crisper way—to make clear to them that their points have gotten across, at least to me.

THERAPIST (*to partners*): Okay, Marie, so you're calling Paul a liar because you're still smarting about his calling you a nag. But, Paul, you're not impressed by that—because you think she *shouldn't* still be smarting.

THERAPIST (*to himself*): Well, I was going for crisp, but it turned out soggy. It's just a repetition of what they themselves said, so I doubt if they got much out of it. I'm sure Casterhazen could have come up with something much better.

MARIE (*looking thoughtful*): Hmm.
PAUL (*looking at Marie*): Hmm.

THERAPIST (*to himself*): But they like it! The tension has disappeared from Marie's face, and Paul has straightened up a bit—he's come out of his discouraged slouch. The fact that they got something from just my simple, soggy repetition shows how deprived of being heard they must have been. They seem to have shifted into the "at-least-Wile-understands-how-I-feel" state of mind. Let's see if I can build on this.

THERAPIST (*to Paul*): You said that Marie *shouldn't* still be smarting. But did it surprise you to hear that she was?

THERAPIST (*to himself*): Paul might feel so bad about having called Marie a nag that he *needs* her to be over it by now—or, even not to have gotten so upset about it in the first place. If so, he might *blame* her for not being over it. He might say something like "It didn't surprise me in the least; Marie holds onto a grudge the way a dog holds onto a bone."

PAUL: I was hoping she wasn't. (*To Marie*) It wasn't the best thing I said last night—calling you a nag. I feel really bad about it.

THERAPIST (*to himself*): Instead of blaming Marie, Paul is admitting things. He has become conciliatory. Let's see if *Marie* follows his lead and becomes conciliatory in return.

MARIE (*to Paul*): Then why did you say it?

THERAPIST (*to himself*): She isn't following his lead.

PAUL: Well, I'll never do it again.
MARIE: I've heard that before.
PAUL: But this time I mean it.
MARIE: That's what you said the last time.

THERAPIST (*to himself*): *That* might explain why Marie didn't follow Paul's lead. She saw what he was doing, not as conciliatory, but as part of an old pattern of contrition, promises, and failure to follow through.

PAUL: But this is different.
MARIE: Talk is cheap.
PAUL: You know, it would help if you had a little faith in me.
MARIE: How can I have faith when you keep breaking your promises?
PAUL: I don't break my promises. I didn't break my promise to wash the dishes every night.

Paul is using Response 2 from the list of defensive responses: **Here's evidence**. But Marie takes exception to Paul's evidence:

MARIE: Sure, if you call leaving half the grease on them "washing" them.
PAUL: (*Shrugs wearily*)

THERAPIST (*to himself*): Both seem clearly displeased with what's happening. Here is one of Cotton's "letups." I'll try what Cotton would say:

THERAPIST (*to partners*): How do you feel about this fight? Are you getting something out of it—a chance to say some things you've been wanting to say, or to hear some things? Or are you just frustrated by it?

It's hard to imagine that Marie and Paul could be getting anything out of this fight. But occasionally partners have surprised me by answering, "It's wonderful—we never get to fight like this at home. I'm saying things I've never been able to say, and I just heard something that really surprised me."

However, this is not one of those times.

MARIE: We've said it all before.
PAUL: Hundreds of times.
MARIE: This could be our living room.
PAUL: It's rehashing old stuff.
MARIE: It's frustrating.
PAUL: How did we get into this?
MARIE: Don't ask me.

THERAPIST (*to himself*): Let's see if I can build a joint platform from which they can look at how they got into this fight.

THERAPIST: Well, maybe we can try to figure it out. When you first came in today, Marie, you said that you've "forgotten that you have a husband." And, at least at that point, there seemed to be a moment of good feeling between the two of you.

MARIE: We had a horrible fight last night. But I realized this morning that it wasn't entirely Paul's fault—in fact, I started it. I burst into the living room—you know how you can open a door in such a way that it sounds the same as slamming it?—and, in my most critical tone of voice, accused Paul of not talking to me any more. So I wanted to use the session today to talk about it in a better way. And, right—as you said—it started out pretty well . . . and then something happened, but I don't know what.

THERAPIST: It seemed to happen at the point when you told Paul it would help if he bathed Jeannie more often.

MARIE: Well, it *would* help.

Marie is defending herself—which suggests that she feels I am accusing her (i.e., that I am saying she *shouldn't* have told Paul about bathing Jeannie).

Things happen fast in a couples therapy session. I want to talk with Marie about whether she feels accused by me, but I realize that I'm not going to get a chance. Marie says to Paul, before I can ask my question:

I should know better than to try to talk about anything serious with you—you always get so defensive.

And now there is another thing I want to talk about: the fact that Marie is accusing Paul. But I know I may not get a chance to do that either. Paul says to Marie:

You're the one who ruined our conversation, you know—by calling me a liar.

I add yet a third item to the list: Paul's defending himself by counterattacking. But, continuing their rapid-fire exchange, Marie says:

Well, you called me a nag.

Here Marie is using Response 15: **I did it only in reaction to what *you* did.**

I am feeling flooded. So instead of following up on any of Marie and Paul's specific comments, I try to talk about what is happening *in general*. I say:

Is *this* an example of what you described a moment ago as "rehashing old stuff" and "being like your living room"?

I am trying to create a "nonadversarial" vantage point from which Marie and Paul can talk about their adversarial interaction. Marie replies:

Well, actually, now that I think about it, I'm *glad* we're talking about this. I wanted a chance to tell Paul how I felt about being called a nag.

Marie is saying that she is getting something out of the fight. And she has joined me on the platform. She is talking in a nonadversarial way about being adversarial. Paul says, however:

But people say a lot of things in a fight that they don't mean. Everyone expects that. No one takes it seriously.

Paul has *not* joined us on the platform. He is continuing to talk in an adversarial way. He is *defending* himself by accusing Marie of overreacting. He is invoking Response 32: **You always make such a big deal about everything.**

MARIE: *No* one takes it seriously? *I* do.
PAUL: Well, you *shouldn't*.

Paul has ratcheted up to a Level 2 attack—"You shouldn't feel what you're feeling." Marie responds:

How do I *know* that you don't mean it seriously? Remember how, in the middle of a fight, you told me that you've always hated my salads? You meant *that* seriously.

Like Paul earlier, Marie is using Response 2: **Here's evidence.**

If Greenholtz were the therapist, he would probably say, "Let's stick to one topic." I prefer, however, to follow along as the partners jump around the board and then, afterwards, try to collect their moves.

- I prefer to track the partners' moment-to-moment reactions rather than to channel those reactions.
- I hesitate to tell partners to stick to one topic, because the topic they are switching to may be more important than the one they are interrupting or may provide crucial new information about the topic they are interrupting.

PAUL: I don't hate your salads—
MARIE: and I'd been making them for *years*.
PAUL: I just said I didn't want one with every meal.
MARIE: Well, why didn't you tell me that before?

Marie is using Response 20: **You should have told me** *sooner.*

PAUL: I didn't want to hurt your feelings.
MARIE: Sure—that's why you won't admit that you think I'm a nag—you "don't want to hurt my feelings."
PAUL: It's not the same thing.
MARIE: How is it different?
PAUL: I was angry. It just slipped out.
MARIE: Yes, it just slipped out. What you *really* felt finally slipped out.

If Greenholtz were the therapist, he would have interrupted this argument long ago. He would see it as an unproductive exchange that, allowed to continue, would simply demoralize Marie and Paul. And Greenholtz is right. So I am planning to interrupt them pretty soon. But I am looking for a way to do so that will not turn me into a traffic cop. I am looking for a way to interrupt them that will tell them something useful about their situation.

PAUL (*wearily*): You don't understand.
MARIE (*looking just as tired*): I understand all right.
PAUL: *You* say things in fights that you don't mean. You called me a liar.
MARIE: What makes you think I didn't mean it?
PAUL: Are you saying you *did* mean it?
MARIE: I don't know any more . . . maybe.
PAUL: Well, *I* didn't mean it when I called you a nag. I only said it in anger.

MARIE: Yes, what you really feel about me finally came out.

Suddenly I think I know how to interrupt their fight in a way that will enable me to say something useful about it. Marie and Paul are stuck: They are going around in circles. What each says contradicts what the other says; that is, neither is able to make his or her point. And that is exactly the point *I* want to make. I say to them:

> Okay, Marie, you're trying to get Paul to admit that he thinks you're a nag. But you're having a hard time doing it—in fact, you're *unable* to do it—because, Paul, *you're* trying to convince Marie that you *don't* think she's a nag. I can understand how the two of you might get pretty frustrated going around and around on this.

I am trying to unstick Marie and Paul by showing them *how* they are stuck and by making their points for them—even if their points are contradictory:

MARIE (*to Paul*): Listen to what this man is saying.
PAUL: I hear him.
MARIE: But do you agree with him?
PAUL: That we're going in circles? Sure.
MARIE: Well, I want to stop.
PAUL: That's fine with me. It wasn't my idea to *start*. I just wanted you to understand that people sometimes say things in fights that they don't mean—like my calling you a nag. I didn't mean it—it just slipped out. I—
MARIE: We've heard all that before—
PAUL: Let me finish. You never let me finish.
MARIE: But I know what you're going to say.

THERAPIST (*to himself*): So do I.

PAUL: No, you don't. It's not what you think it is. If you'd let me finish, you'll see that it's different.
MARIE: Well, it started out the same—
PAUL: Just let me *finish*.
MARIE: Okay, okay.

Actually, it *was* going to be the same. But since Paul has insisted it was going to be different, he has to *make* it appear different. He can't think of anything new to say about the "nag" issue, but he *can* say something different about Marie's calling him a liar.

PAUL: All right, maybe I *didn't* bathe Jeannie last week. Maybe it was the week before. But it was an honest mistake. I got the weeks confused, that's all. I'm not a *liar*.

THERAPIST (*to himself*): This really *is* different. I'm surprised.

MARIE: Well, I'm tired of your "honest" mistakes. If they're so honest, why do you keep making them? I—
PAUL (*interrupting*): Yes, but—
MARIE (*interrupting Paul's interruption*): Let me finish. I didn't interrupt you when you were talking.
PAUL: Yes, but—
MARIE: I didn't interrupt *you*.
PAUL (*reluctantly*): All right. Go on.
MARIE: As I was saying before I was interrupted, I'm tired of your "honest" mistakes. Saying that you bathed Jeannie last week is just the latest in a long string. And, frankly, your mistakes don't always look "honest" to me. They always somehow make you look good—and you *do* look good. My mother and sister are convinced you're the perfect husband. You fool everybody. Okay, maybe it's true that you do more around the house than most husbands we know, but it's still always up to me to organize things, to initiate things, to make sure things get done, including making sure *you* get certain things done—which sometimes puts me in a position of what you so endearingly call a nag. The point is, when it comes down to it, everything's really up to me. And I feel really lonely—maybe that's the *real* point—I feel so . . . lonely.
PAUL: Are you finished?
MARIE: Yes.
PAUL: Well, I don't understand why you even want me to bathe Jeannie. You don't like the way I do it. You hover over me giving me instructions.

THERAPIST (*to himself*): Marie isn't going to like it that Paul ignored what she said. And she won't like the word "hover" either.

MARIE: I *don't* hover.
PAUL: First you come in and tell me that the water's too cold. Then you tell me I'm using the wrong powder. What would *you* call it if not hovering?
MARIE: I haven't done anything like that in months. You don't give me credit for trying to change.

THERAPIST (*to himself*): Important things are being said here but they're getting buried. Let's see if I can dig them out.

THERAPIST (*to partners*): There's a conversation hidden within your fight, but it's easy to miss *because* of the fight. So let me interrupt the fight for a moment and try to find the conversation.

THERAPIST (*to himself*): I've got their interest. Paul just straightened up in his chair again and Marie is looking at me. They're probably wondering what possible conversation I see hidden in their fight.

THERAPIST (*to partners*): Paul, you're saying to Marie, "You're right, I didn't bathe Jeannie last week; it was 2 weeks ago. But I'm afraid to admit it because I'm worried you're going to say, 'See, see, I told you you were a liar!'" And Marie, you're saying, "Yes, well how *else* can I see it?" And Paul, you're saying, "Well, you could see it as a mistake—an honest mistake." And Marie, you're saying, "Yes, but that's not even the point—in fact, I just figured out what the point is. It's that I feel *lonely*, that all the organizing and arranging are up to me. *That's* what I want you to see: that I feel *lonely*." (*To Marie*) Am I overstating it?

MARIE: You're *under*stating it. That's the crux of the matter. I feel *lonely*.

THERAPIST: And Paul, you're saying, "I never know what to do when you say things like this—you know, that you feel lonely. I feel bad—that I've done something wrong, that I've let you down. I can't think of what to say, so I wind up not saying anything." (*To Paul*) I know you didn't exactly say this. I'm making it up. You can tell me if I'm wrong.

PAUL: Well, it is those things, but it's also that I feel like a failure as a husband.

THERAPIST (*to himself*): That's a shocker—Paul is admitting even more than I admitted *for* him.

THERAPIST (*to partners*): Okay, so you're saying, "I feel like a failure as a husband. And, besides, I don't know that you really want my help. You never like the way I do things. I've got my way of bathing Jeannie, but you want me to do it *your* way. And I feel hurt and discounted and angry and like saying, 'Fine, then, *you* do it.'" And Marie, you're saying—or at least I think you're saying—"Yes, I know you think I interfere when you bathe Jeannie—so I've been trying to hold my tongue and let you do it your way. And *I* feel hurt and discounted and angry that you haven't noticed the change."

THERAPIST (*to himself*): That came out well. Casterhazen couldn't have said it better—although I've got to remember to get back to Paul's comment about feeling like a failure as a husband. That sounded pretty important.

My purpose here is not to teach Marie and Paul how to communicate, although they may easily misunderstand what I am saying as such. I am trying to give them a new way to think and a new way to have a relationship:

> I want them to know, when they shoot their quills at each other, that each has a soft underbelly (e.g., "I feel lonely," "I feel like a failure as a husband")—even if at the moment they're unable to pick out what it is.
>
> I want them to know that when they have a fight, there is a conversation hidden within it—even if they have no idea where it is or how to look for it.
>
> I want them to know that there is a collaborative way to talk about the issues they are fighting about—even if they cannot figure out what it is.
>
> I want them to know that there is a way to understand what is happening to them—even if, at the moment, the situation seems chaotic and to make no sense at all.
>
> I want them to know that both of them are in a difficult situation: struggling to get something important across to the other that they have yet to fully figure out.

As I have said, Marie and Paul may easily misunderstand what I am saying as simply teaching them how to talk. This misunderstanding may be furthered by the fact that, in digging out the conversation buried in their fight, I am using what is perhaps the major principle of good communication: making "I statements" rather than "you statements." The conversation that I make up for Marie and Paul consists essentially of a string of "I statements."

But the heart of what I am doing is not simply obeying a rule: "making 'I statements' instead of 'you statements.'" I am trying to set the relationship on a new footing by creating a joint platform.

Making up this dialogue for Marie and Paul requires some guesses on my part. In some cases these guesses are easy to make. When Marie says, "I haven't done anything like that in months" (i.e., interfered when Paul bathed Jeannie), it is easy to infer an "I statement": "Yes, I know you feel I interfere when you bathe Jeannie—that's why I've been trying not to interfere. And I'm disappointed that you haven't noticed the change."

At other times, I infer the "I statement" from what I know about the partners—in particular, what they have told me in previous sessions or earlier in the hour. Paul mentioned two sessions before that he feels hurt when Marie disapproves of the way he takes care of the kids.

At still other times, I make guesses based on what I have heard others say in similar situations. It is not difficult to guess that Paul deals with his hurt by saying to himself, "If Marie doesn't like the way I bathe Jeannie, fine; *she* can do it."

In guessing a partner's "I statements," I try not to go farther than the partners themselves feel comfortable going; that is, I try to avoid suggesting feelings that a partner might experience as accusing, humiliating, or undercutting. I say for Paul, "I never know what to do when you say you feel lonely; I feel bad—that I've done something wrong, that I've let you down," because I feel that chances are good that Paul will welcome this rather than wince at my saying this for him.

As time goes on, I find myself increasingly better at discovering the "I statements" hidden in partners' "you statements." And when I guess wrong, I can generally count on the partners to correct me (I ask them to correct me). Even my wrong guesses are helpful, since they typically stimulate the partners to make their own more accurate "I statements."

My hope is that Marie and Paul will respond to my revealing the conversation hidden within their fight by saying, "I wish *we* could have said it that way." For a moment at least, they will then be on a joint platform looking down at the fight. But Marie says:

I'm tired of being the only one who can talk like that.

I have been hoping to show Marie and Paul how, even in the middle of a fight, there is a conversation going on. But my comments have just reminded Marie of her resentment at Paul for *not* talking in the way I have just done for the two of them. Paul responds:

Who *says* you talk like that?

Paul is using Response 12 (**You do the same thing**)—that is, You're no better at it than I am—which Marie rebuts as follows:

MARIE: Well, I *used* to talk like that—before I got so frustrated that I gave up trying.

PAUL: You always think you're so perfect—so high and mighty. I can't stand how self-righteous you get.

MARIE: Well, *I* can't stand the thought of spending the rest of my life with a man who has no answers, no questions, and never anything to say to me.

THERAPIST (*to himself*): That could flatten Paul.

PAUL: You knew I wasn't much of a talker when you married me.

Paul is using Response 22: **You knew what you were getting, so you have only yourself to blame.**

Marie and Paul are using my statement as ammunition in their ongoing battle with each other. Instead of using it to create a joint platform, they are incorporating it into their fight. Fortunately, I am used to this—which is good, since otherwise I could easily get frustrated and start blaming Marie and Paul (for being resistant) or myself (for giving them the additional ammunition).

Marie and Paul seem so dedicated to the fight—so caught up in it—that it's easy to forget that fighting is a fallback position. It's a consolation prize. In a fight—in fact, this is the definition of a fight—the fighters give up trying to reason with each other and, instead, try to:

> Punish the other person in an effort to compensate for the injury they feel has been done to them.

> Bully or browbeat the other person in an effort to force him or her to listen, submit, comply, change—or to admit his or her error, guilt, or failing.

The other person typically responds by digging in his or her heels. Fighting is a fallback position in which the new goal (punishing the other) makes it less likely that the person will accomplish the original goal, which is to get the other person to listen. That is why Marie and Paul's fight is unresolvable: Neither is able to get the other to acknowledge any of his or her points.

Alice Eberheart (the radio-show therapist mentioned in Chapter 6), who sees all behavior as serving a purpose, would see Marie and Paul as unwilling to stop their fight because they are getting too much out of it. "Fighting is their way of establishing contact and enlivening their relationship," she would say; "it serves a purpose." But where Eberheart would see Marie and Paul as getting too *much* out of their fight to be willing to stop, I see them as getting too *little* out of it to be able to stop. Neither is getting the crucial satisfaction of feeling the other is listening.

One way to end the fight, accordingly, is by helping Marie and Paul state their points in a way that will enable the other to listen. Paul has just replied to Marie's "*I* can't stand the thought of spending the rest of my life with a man who has no answers, no questions, and never anything to say to me," by saying, "You knew I wasn't much of a talker when you married me." So I try to make a statement for Paul that Marie *may* be able to listen to—and, at the same time, that may enable Paul to express more fully what he feels:

Paul, you must feel *devastated* hearing what Marie just said.

Paul may flinch at this. "Devastated" is a strong word. But I *need* a strong word, so I take the chance. He replies:

> That's too strong. I don't feel "devastated" . . . it's more that I feel . . . well, actually, maybe that *is* what I feel—devastated. In fact, that's *exactly* what I feel.

"Devastated" is not a word that Paul would ordinarily think to use. In fact, he first fights it off. It makes him nervous. But once he adjusts to it, he appears to enjoy my using it.

The word has an immediate and powerful impact on Marie. She says to Paul:

> Well, I didn't want you to feel *devastated* . . . Shaken up, maybe. Well, all right, just a *little* devastated—but I didn't want to *really* hurt you. I know I get pretty harsh sometimes.

Marie has snapped into the "I-feel-bad-about-what-I-said" state. She is being conciliatory. But Paul replies:

> You're not harsh—"harsh" is what cleansers are. What you are is a menace.

I say to myself:

> What's wrong with Paul? Marie just made a conciliatory comment. Instead of returning the favor, he's using what she said against her. Why did he have to go and do that? He's being totally unreasonable. Here I make my best effort to get a good conversation going—and I'm succeeding—and they seem to be enjoying it—and, then, pow, on one statement, Paul destroys it all. He must have a narcissistic character disorder. Oops, careful, Wile. Don't look now, but you've shifted from analyzing to judging. You've fallen off the platform. It's good that you realized that before you said anything.

To get back *on* the platform—that is, to shift from judging Paul to appreciating the situation he is dealing with—I look to see whether Paul's seemingly inappropriate response may be appropriate to the immediate situation in a way that is not immediately obvious—that is, to something going on in the relationship (or to an anticipated reaction from Marie) that may make his response understandable. And I look to see how his behavior may be a consequence of his inability to formulate and articulate this concern.

To check out these possibilities, I say:

> Paul, Marie appeared to be feeling conciliatory. She told you that she felt bad about what she said. But you didn't take it as a peace offering. So either Marie *was* conciliatory but you didn't see it—or *I* missed something and she really wasn't conciliatory, or not conciliatory enough—or it was too little too late—or you thought she was trying to get off easy—or you hadn't yet gotten over what she said earlier—or something else entirely.

Why don't I simply ask Paul, "Why did you react to Marie's conciliatory remark by becoming nonconciliatory?" and leave it at that? Because I feel that Paul (or anyone in his position) may experience such a question as a reproach—that what I really am saying is that he *should* have been conciliatory. So I need to show him that my question is *not* a reproach. And my way to do this is to ask the question and then suggest possible answers—answers making it clear that I assume he has good reason for being nonconciliatory (i.e., that his nonconciliatory response makes sense)—and it is just a matter of our figuring out what his reason is.

And Paul's response makes it clear that he does *not* feel reproached by me:

PAUL: What Marie said was okay—*in itself*. I was just worried what she was going to say *next*—because *that's* what's been happening this whole hour: She starts by saying something nice and then—pow!—she lets me have it.

THERAPIST (*to himself*): Hmm, I guess he's right.

PAUL (*continuing*): And I've been doing the same to her.

THERAPIST (*to himself*): What a crucial addition! Paul is being conciliatory in the very act of explaining his being *non*conciliatory.

MARIE: It's been a pretty shaky hour, all right.

For a moment Marie and Paul are on the joint platform. They are talking noncombatively about their argument.

I look at the clock—only 5 minutes left. When clients notice my looking at the clock, they probably think I am hoping the hour will end soon. They don't realize that I am more likely hoping the hour will *not* end soon—so that we will have time:

- To get to what we need to.
- To follow up on all the loose ends.
- Or, if the session is going poorly, to give it a chance to turn around.

THERAPIST: I remember you said last time that when a session doesn't go
   well, it ruins the rest of the evening. Is that going to happen tonight?
PAUL: It's going to be pretty quiet on the way home.
MARIE: I'm just glad we have a radio in the car.

When it looks to me as if partners are going to leave the session
upset with each other or unhappy about what happened in the session,
I try to create a "nonangry" vantage point from which they can talk about
how the coming evening (or week) is likely to turn out as a result of
the session.

THERAPIST: And when you get home, then?
MARIE: We'll each do our own thing.
PAUL: We probably won't even see one another until it's time to put the
   kids to bed.
MARIE: And we'll just talk to them, not each other.

Marie and Paul are talking collaboratively about how noncollabora-
tive they are going to be.

THERAPIST: And after the kids are in bed—?
PAUL: I'll probably watch TV.
MARIE: I have some reports to finish.
PAUL: It's going to be pretty quiet.
MARIE: It's going to be pretty *lonely*.

THERAPIST (*to himself*): There's that "lonely" again.

THERAPIST (*to partners*): And in this quiet and lonely evening, will there
   be a moment when either of you feels at least a little tempted to
   try to say something to the other?
PAUL: Not me—I'm down for the count.
MARIE: I wouldn't know what to say.
THERAPIST: What about what you just said here—that you feel lonely?
MARIE: But Paul would just shrug and I'd feel like a fool for opening my
   mouth.
THERAPIST (*to Paul*): Is that what you'd do, shrug and say nothing?
PAUL: Probably.
THERAPIST: And that's because—?
PAUL: —because the next thing Marie would say is "Why do *I* always
   have to be the one who makes the first move? Why can't *you* take
   the initiative once in a while?" And I don't want to give her the
   chance.
THERAPIST (*to Paul*): Oh, it's like what you just said: You'd see Marie as

doing something nice—reaching out, making the first move—and then, wham, she'd attack.

MARIE (*to Paul*): Is that why you don't answer me, because you think I'm going to attack you?

PAUL: Why do you think?

MARIE: I think you're just being your usual tight-lipped self.

PAUL: What do you think *makes* me my usual tight-lipped self?

THERAPIST (*to himself, looking again at the clock*): Oh-oh. We're already 2 minutes *over* the hour, but it's a bad time to stop: Marie and Paul have just resumed their fight. Let's see if I can produce some semblance of closure.

THERAPIST (*to partners*): We need to stop—but, Marie, maybe the main thing you've been trying to get Paul to see is that you feel *lonely*, particularly when he's quiet, but you haven't found a way to tell him this without his feeling attacked.

MARIE: I don't think there *is* a way.

THERAPIST: And, Paul, maybe the main thing you've been trying to get Marie to see is that you feel *attacked*, and *that's* one of the major reasons you get quiet.

PAUL: Well, yes, I—

MARIE (*interrupting*): But what can we *do* about it?

THERAPIST (*to himself*): *That's* the problem with closing summaries. Sometimes they open things instead of close them. But it's too late to take this any further.

THERAPIST (*to partners*): We've run out of time. So, for the moment, we'll have to leave that hanging. We can talk about it next week . . . I'll see you then.

Marie and Paul say goodbye and leave my office. I say to myself:

Robert Langs would disapprove. I went 5 minutes over—he'd see me as violating the frame. Of course, I don't know what Langs's opinion is of couples therapy—he might see *that* as violating the frame. So I might as well just forget about Langs.

I sit down to write down a few summary words.

My Notes

Marie feels lonely, in part because Paul doesn't talk; Paul feels criticized—that's partly why he doesn't talk. When I told them that, Marie said, "But what can we do about it?"

Marie also feels lonely because although Paul behaves in ways that make him look good to the outside world, it's still really all up to her—all the organizing, initiating, making up after fights.

Paul feels criticized, but he's also worried about *criticizing* (as I now realize while writing these notes). He suppressed his complaint about the salads, and he tried to convince Marie that he doesn't see her as a nag. She wasn't convinced, however.

They said the session was going to ruin their evening.

I file these notes, review my notes on the couple I am about to see, and head for the waiting room to usher them in. Halfway down the hall, I stop, rush back to my office, recover my notes on Marie and Paul, and pencil in at the bottom: "Paul said at one point that he feels like a failure as a husband—but I forgot to follow up on this."

Why do I go to all the trouble to correct an omission? Because writing these notes—or, rather, reading them just before Marie and Paul's next session—turns me into a sharper therapist. And the more complete the notes, the better. *Without* these notes, I would listen to Marie and Paul with only a vague memory of what happened the previous session. *With* these notes, I will listen to Marie and Paul with the following in mind:

Questions I Have at My Fingertips
as a Result of Having Just Reviewed My Notes

1. Did you have the quiet and lonely evening after last week's session that you expected?
2. What do you think about the idea from last time that you, Marie, feel lonely and that you, Paul, feel attacked?
3. And what do you think of the idea, Paul (it occurred to me after the session) that in addition to feeling attacked, you are also concerned about *attacking*—or about Marie's seeing you as attacking? You tried to convince her that you *don't* think she is a nag.
4. And where are you on that issue this week—Paul, your belief that you don't see Marie as a nag and, Marie, your belief that he does?
5. Have you had any further thoughts about Marie's feeling that Paul does things to make himself look good but it's still mostly up to Marie—all the arranging, the making sure things get done, and the reaching out after fights?
6. Paul, you mentioned last week that you felt like a failure as a husband. Was that something that you just felt at that moment or something you feel a lot?

I don't write down these questions—I don't have to. They are implicit in my notes. All I have to do is read the notes and the questions pop into my mind. I don't always ask all of them—or even any of them—since new issues often arise that take precedence. But I have these questions at my fingertips if I do wish to ask them.

The Next Session

At the next session, Marie and Paul come in and say:

PAUL: Guess what? We didn't have any fights this week.
MARIE: But don't get too excited—that's just because we've been so busy.
PAUL: There wasn't *time* to fight—in fact, we hardly had a chance to talk at all.
MARIE: So it's been a pretty good week.

Having just reviewed my notes, I am able to say:

THERAPIST (*to Marie*): Going by what we said last week, Marie, "hardly having a chance to talk to each other" *wouldn't* make it a "pretty good week"—because, as you said, you feel *lonely* when you and Paul don't talk.
MARIE: I don't understand it either. Somehow it was a good week even if we didn't talk.
PAUL (*to Marie*): But we *did* talk. Don't you remember? We had a long talk after leaving here—and another one a couple of days ago.
MARIE: Well, yes, now that you mention it . . .

Having just reviewed my notes, I say:

THERAPIST: So you *didn't* have the quiet and lonely evening after last time that you thought you'd have.
PAUL: We had the *best* conversation we've had in months—although I don't remember much about it.
MARIE: Me neither.
THERAPIST: What *do* you remember?
PAUL: We were in the car. Marie turned off the radio and asked me if I really meant it when I said—you know, what I said last time about feeling "inadequate"—no, that's not it—it was something *like* that.
MARIE: I don't remember either.

Having just read my notes, *I* remember:

THERAPIST (*to Paul*): You said you felt like a failure as a husband.
PAUL: Yes, *that's* it.

MARIE (*to Paul*): It shocked me to hear it. You always seem so above it all. It's hard to imagine you feeling like a failure as a husband.

PAUL: When you tell me I let you down, I take it to heart.

MARIE: Well, you'd never know it. You never seem to listen to *anything* I say.

THERAPIST (*to himself*): I don't think Paul's going to like that.

MARIE (*continuing*): Of course, you may feel that I never listen to *you* either—especially when we fight the way we did last session.

THERAPIST (*to himself*): Back from the brink.

PAUL: That's why I was so surprised when you asked me if I really felt like a failure as a husband. I didn't think you'd *care* after all the angry stuff we said to each other.

MARIE: Well, I got some things off my chest. I got to say that I felt lonely. I don't know whether you heard it, but at least I got to say it.

PAUL: I heard it: Why do you think I felt like a failure as a husband?

Getting to say that she felt lonely, even if she was unsure whether Paul heard it, was all Marie needed to be able to begin to listen to him. Getting to say that he felt like a failure as a husband and feeling that Marie heard him were all Paul needed to begin listening to her. And feeling that Paul *was* listening to her was all Marie needed to feel less lonely, to feel better about him, and to have a better week.

And now we have a clearer idea of the crucial points that Marie and Paul suffered from being unable to make in the previous session. Marie got upset and started fighting when she was unable to tell Paul that she felt lonely in the relationship. Paul got upset and started fighting when he was unable to tell Marie that he felt like a failure as a husband.

Conclusion

At any given moment in a couples therapy session, I look for the points that the partners need to make. And then I look for the points they need to make next—and the moment after that and the moment after that. I do this primarily by:

1. *Interviewing*—for example, by asking, "Marie, what do you feel at the moment?"

2. *Suggesting possible answers*—for example, by saying, "Do you feel frustrated? Sad? Discouraged? Angry?"

3. *Making their points for them* (saying crisply what each person has said in a vague and roundabout way; that is, uncovering the "I message"

hidden in the person's "you message")—for example, by saying, "Okay, Marie, so you're saying in essence: 'When Paul comes home and doesn't talk to me as much as I'd like, I feel *lonely.*'"

4. *Helping the other partner formulate a response*—for example, by saying, "Okay, Paul, so when Marie says she feels lonely, you feel like a failure as a husband."

5. *Finding the logjam* (showing that a particular argument is unresolvable, because the point that each partner is trying to make conflicts with the point that the other partner is trying to make)—for example, by saying, "Okay, Marie, you're trying to get Paul to admit that he thinks you're a nag. But you're having a hard time doing it—in fact, you're *unable* to do it—because, Paul, *you're* trying to convince Marie that you *don't* think she's a nag. I can understand how the two of you might get pretty frustrated going around and around on this."

6. *Constructing a dialogue* (revealing the conversation hidden in the partners' fight)—for example, by saying, "Okay, Paul, so you're saying in essence. . . . And in reply, Marie, you're saying in essence. . . . And in reply to that, Paul, you're saying in essence. . . ."

Why is it so important to help partners make their points?

• *Because the partners' inability to make their points is what maintains the fight.* It is what makes a fight unresolvable. That is the main point of this *chapter* (and the other chapters on couple fighting): to show that fighting is a fallback position; it is what partners do when they are unable to make their points.

• *Because the partners' inability to make their points lies at the root of their problems.* That is a major point of this *book*. The moment-by-moment account of Marie and Paul's evening reveals how their inability to say, or even to know, what is on their minds—that is, to make their points—is the principal source of their problems.

CHAPTER 15

The Shifting In and Out
of an Adversarial State
between Client and Therapist

As shown throughout this book, Marie and Paul—and, by extension, couples in general—shift in and out of adversarial states. These states take the form of cutting looks, angry or withdrawn silences, innuendo, sarcastic asides, grumpiness, whining, sulking, shrugs, raised eyebrows, raised voices, exaggerated indictments, ultimatums, slamming of doors, and (in some couples) physical abuse.

Similarly, there is a continuous shifting in and out of a subtle (and sometimes not so subtle) adversarial tone between the therapist and the client—and, in couples therapy, between the therapist and one or both partners.

True, couples therapists are less likely than their clients to become accusing and defensive. Unlike Marie and Paul, I *don't* have my partner sitting next to me criticizing me or refusing to listen as I criticize her. Even so, as this book reveals, it's easy for me, like my clients, to become accusing or defensive without knowing it (since for me also, part of fighting is thinking that I am not fighting). Of course, *realizing* how easy it is to fight without knowing it gives me a leg up on recognizing when it happens.

As I recommend for people in relating to their partners, I have tried to become increasingly skillful in:

1. Tracking the shifting in and out of an adversarial tone between me and my clients.
2. Anticipating which interventions are likely to provoke the clients' defensiveness, counteraccusations, or discouragement.

3. Using my clients' defensiveness and accusations as a clue that I may just now have been unwittingly defensive or accusing.
4. Appreciating the inevitability of my becoming accusing or defensive without knowing it—in other words, becoming increasingly better at recognizing it, at least after the fact.
5. Not being thrown by the realization that I have been adversarial (accusing or defensive) with my clients.

This fifth item is the key to the others. To the extent that I become less derailed and more forgiving toward myself for being adversarial with my clients, I will be able to do the first four things on the list: track, anticipate, pick up clues, and appreciate the inevitability of my becoming adversarial. If I do *not* forgive myself, I am likely to block out the discomforting awareness that I am being adversarial. Self-forgiveness is, in this instance, a prerequisite for awareness.

But why is it that I become unknowingly accusing or defensive with my clients? The answer lies in the early chapters of this book. Marie has been our stand-in. I have described how she, and thus by extension all of us (clients *and* therapists), are at certain crucial times:

Just a step ahead of our harsh internal taskmaster.
On the verge of feeling that we are doing or feeling something wrong.
Struggling to justify our reactions.
Snapping out moral injunctions to counter our harsh internal taskmaster's moral injunctions.
Dealing with our partners in the same way our taskmaster deals with us.

How does this explain why I and other therapists become unwittingly accusing and defensive with their clients? The answer is that this "looking-over-our-shoulders, worrying-about-being-jumped, self-suspicious, harsh-internal-taskmaster-dominated" thinking pervades our lives—and our language. Much of what we think, say, and do contains a hidden or not-so-hidden reproach: a "shaking-of-the-finger, slap-on-the-wrist, should-or-shouldn't" tone.

We talk about people being "courageous"—about their "willingness to take risks"—and that sounds like a good thing. But implicit in such statements is the idea that *other* people (or even these same people at other times) are cowardly and unwilling to take risks.
We tell people that they are "dependent" or "codependent," and we think we are giving them information that is useful—that will give

them the option of behaving differently. And sometimes it does. But if they find it difficult to behave differently, they might now be burdened with the self-hating thought: "I'm being dependent" or "I'm being codependent."

How can we tell whether a particular comment has a moralistic, "shaking-of-the-finger" tone? Easy—all we have to do is to notice whether the words "You should" or "You shouldn't" are implied. (Another test is to judge whether or not we would want such a comment made about us.)

> When we say, "You're a workaholic," what we really mean is "You shouldn't be a workaholic; it's self-destructive to be a workaholic."
> When we say, "You're late," what we really mean is "You shouldn't be late; it's rude to be late."
> When we say, "You're running away from your problems," what we really mean is "You should face them."
> When we say, "You're trying to make me feel guilty," we're saying, "It's not right to make someone feel guilty."
> When we say, "Isn't it about time that you finally forgave your parents?", we are saying, "You should have already done it by now."

Certain classic psychotherapeutic interventions have such a "should-or-shouldn't" cast to them:

1. The intervention "You are trying to control the hour" is hard for clients to hear without feeling they are being told, "You *shouldn't* try to control the hour."
2. The intervention "You're resisting" is hard for clients to hear without feeling they are being told that resisting is bad.
3. The intervention "You bring up issues at the end of the hour when we won't be able to talk about them" is hard for clients to hear without feeling that they are being reprimanded for not bringing up issues earlier in the hour, when there *was* time to talk about them.

Similarly:

4. "You want me magically to solve your problems" is easily heard as "At your age you shouldn't believe in magicians."
5. "You haven't mentioned your coming 5 minutes late today" can

be heard as "You *should* have mentioned it," or even "You should be on time."

6. "You're angry" can be heard as "Anger is not an appropriate response."
7. "You're afraid of anger" can be heard as "You *shouldn't* be afraid of it."
8. "The anger you're expressing toward me is really anger at your father" (or "You're angry at me as you were angry at your father long ago") can be heard as "Your anger at me is unjustified."
9. "You see me siding with your husband the same way as you felt your mother favored your brother" can be heard as "Your grievance with me is misplaced."
10. "Say it to him (her), not to me" can be heard as "You *should* have said it to him (her) in the first place."
11. "That's a 'you statement'" can be heard as "Only 'I statements' are accepted here."

Am I criticizing these 11 classic psychotherapeutic interventions and the therapists who make them? Am I saying that therapists should *not* make interventions that imply "should"? Am I being judgmental about these therapists' being judgmental?

Yes.

As I see it, everyone's basic problem is self-reproach (shame, guilt, self-blame, self-hate, negative self-talk, the punitive superego, the harsh internal taskmaster) and, more generally, feeling unentitled to certain feelings. My therapeutic goal is to establish a vantage point from which clients can observe the existence, effects of, and reactions to their sense of unentitlement to their feelings and to their "moralizing, harsh-internal-taskmaster-dominated, should-and-shouldn't-oriented" thinking. I thus try to avoid interventions (such as the 11 listed above) that reinforce the client's "should-and-shouldn't-oriented" thinking.

Some may wonder whether my effort to avoid reinforcing clients' self-reproach prevents me from confronting clients with important but painful truths about themselves. As I see it, clients are *already* confronting themselves with painful "truths"—for example, they are criticizing themselves for being "codependent," afraid of intimacy," or "narcissistic." And *that* is the problem: this self-reproach and their effort to defend themselves against it.

Of course, my whole approach arises from my assumption that much of the problem is the "shoulds and shouldn'ts" with which people are already burdened. If I had a different theory, I would have a different attitude toward these 11 common interventions.

Let us say that I were to have the "therapy-is-essentially-resistance-analysis" theory. I would believe that:

> The most crucial fact about the client is that he or she is in a state of resistance.
>
> The main thing going on at any given moment in a therapy session is that the client is defending against threatening awarenesses, resisting positive change, rebelling against the therapist's authority, trying to sabotage the therapy, and/or trying to fulfill regressive wishes rather than analyze them.
>
> Therapy, then, consists essentially of confronting these defenses and resistances by interpreting them.

If I were to have this view, I wouldn't think of it as judgmental to tell clients "You're resisting" (Item 2 on the numbered list above) or "You bring up issues at the end of the hour so we won't be able to talk about them" (Item 3). I would think of it as doing my job.

Given the view I *do* have, I don't see it as much of a problem that the client brings up an issue at the end of the hour, when there is no time to discuss it. The client *has* brought it up, after all, and I can easily reintroduce the issue in the next session, when there *is* time to discuss it. To a therapist with the "therapy-is-essentially-resistance-analysis" perspective, however, I would be missing the point, which is not just to finesse resistance but to confront it—to bring to the client's awareness the fact that he or she is resisting.

Here is another example. Let us say that I were to have the "therapy-is-essentially-resisting-the-client's-dependency-pulls" theory (in contrast to the "people-suffer-from-self-reproaches-and-feeling-unentitled-to-feelings" theory that I do have). I would believe that:

> Clients try to seduce you into taking over their lives (use you as a crutch, become dependent on you) rather than taking responsibility for themselves.
>
> It is crucial, therefore, not to play into the client's dependency pulls (therapy becomes possible only to the extent that you don't).
>
> What is needed to set the therapy on its proper course is to make clear that the change is going to come from the client and not from the therapist.

Were I to have this view, I wouldn't see it as judgmental (as fostering "should-and-shouldn't-oriented" thinking) to tell clients, "You want me magically to solve your problems" (Item 4 on the numbered list). In fact, I would see therapists who did not confront their clients' dependency pulls in this way as shrinking from their responsibility.

Here is a third and final example. Let us say that I were to have the "using-the-transference-to-trace-the-problem-to-childhood" theory of therapy. If I were to have this view, I wouldn't see it as judgmental to tell clients, "Your anger at me is like your anger at your father long ago." I would see it, in fact, as the crucial point to make.

How a therapist views the 11 interventions on the list is a function of his or her theory. Whereas I see these interventions as pejorative, judgmental, adversarial, and departing from neutrality, therapists working from different perspectives see them as objective, neutral, and what therapy is all about.

As I have said, my particular theory, which leads to my attitude toward these 11 interventions, is based on the idea that people suffer primarily from self-reproach—and, more generally, from feeling unentitled to feelings. As a therapist I will inevitably at times arouse the client's harsh internal taskmaster despite my best efforts. In response, the client may become subtly or overtly adversarial (i.e., defensive or accusing). In turn, I may become subtly adversarial without knowing it. Therapy consists of an inevitable shifting in and out of an adversarial state between the therapist and the client.

CHAPTER 16

Monitoring the Shifting In and Out of an Adversarial State between Client and Therapist

The fine-grained analysis of Marie and Paul's evening presented in this book produces a picture of how people:

Catapult through a continuous series of half-thoughts and half-feelings.

Struggle with anxiety and with their harsh internal taskmaster.

Ratchet through a continuous series of mental states and, with their partners, a continuous series of couple states.

Pass through these mental states, in part in an attempt to deal with their harsh internal taskmaster.

Are caught up in an interpersonal atmosphere that is formed in part by the effect of everyone else's harsh internal taskmaster.

Whether or not a client experiences a therapist's intervention as accusatory depends to an important extent on the client's state of mind. If I say to Paul, "You look angry,"

And if Paul replies, "You can say that again," I take it as evidence that he is in the "feeling-it's-okay-to-be-angry" state of mind.

But if Paul replies, "I'm not angry; I'm just puzzled," I take it as evidence that he is in the "feeling-rebuked-by-the-harsh-internal-taskmaster-for-feeling-angry, feeling-the-provocation-is-insufficient-to-justify-feeling-angry" state of mind. (Of course, it is also possible that, exactly as he says, he is *not* feeling angry at all.)

If Paul is in the "feeling-it's-not-okay-to-be-angry" state of mind, my "You look angry" is likely to provoke his defensiveness; that is, he is likely to experience my comment as accusing. We typically think of defensiveness as a characteristic of the client—which it is. *But defensiveness is also a function of the therapist*: It is a consequence of the therapist's failure to take into account the client's state of mind when making an interpretation. If I say, "You look angry,"

> What I *mean* is this: "Anger is a part of life; everyone continually goes in and out of it. In fact, anger is useful. It's a clue to something important going on in the relationship. That's why I'm asking you about it now."
>
> What Paul *hears*, however, is this: "I'm onto you. You're angry. Admit it. And you *shouldn't* be angry. There's no justification for it. You're overreacting. It's weak, immature, and unmanly to be angry just because Marie complains about your not taking the initiative."

In other words, Paul hears my "You look angry" through the mediating voice of his harsh internal taskmaster. And hearing it through this voice, he becomes defensive:

> I'm not angry. I'm just puzzled.

Which means that Paul has snapped into the "narrowed-down, protecting-myself-from-Wile-and-from-my-harsh-internal-taskmaster" state of mind, and he has lost his ability to think and to collaborate. To keep this from happening, I do *not* say, "You look angry." Instead, I tell him:

> "Given what just happened, Paul, I imagine that you might feel frustrated" (or "exasperated" or "fed up"). I choose a synonym for "angry" that I believe will not provoke the taskmaster's moral recriminations.
>
> Or "Most people would feel angry in this situation. Do you?" Paul's harsh internal taskmaster tells him that he should not feel angry unless there is clear and present cause. So I suggest that there is sufficient cause, and that *most* people would feel angry in his situation.
>
> Or "I imagine you could be feeling disappointed or discouraged or frustrated or angry." By listing "angry" as only one of several possibilities, I am making it less identifiable as a feeling for which Paul thinks I am reproaching him.

My goal is not just to elude Paul's taskmaster, but to create a platform from which Paul can become aware of this taskmaster—that is, his internal recriminations. With this in mind, I say:

> I get the idea that you feel you *shouldn't* feel angry unless you can justify it by pointing to a clear and present provocation.

I am trying to create a "nonjudgmental" vantage point from which Paul can notice his judgmental thinking (his "shouldn't"). Instead of looking relieved, however, he appears even more burdened.

THERAPIST: You seem discouraged by what I just said.
PAUL: I should know by now that a feeling is its own justification. I shouldn't need you to remind me.

This means that, without missing a beat, Paul's harsh internal taskmaster has shifted from one rebuke ("You shouldn't feel angry; you don't have justification") to another ("You should know by now that anger is its own justification"). It is clear that I have *not* established a platform— a "nonrebuking" position—from which Paul can view his internal rebukes. Paul's internal voice has co-opted my comment and turned it into a new moral recrimination.

As this example shows, it can be difficult at times to create a platform from which the client can become aware of his or her internal taskmaster. So I try to create a platform from which Paul can appreciate the difficulty of creating such a platform. I suggest to Paul that he may be in a state of mind—a common one for all of us—in which everything becomes material for self-accusation. I realize, of course, given Paul's state of mind, that he may also hear *this* comment as a criticism. In other words, I know that my attempt may fail once again to create a "nonself-criticizing" vantage point from which he can look at his self-criticizing.

Whenever a client becomes defensive, I immediately consider the possibility that I have become reproaching without knowing it—that I have aligned myself with the client's taskmaster. This rule of thumb I have for myself parallels the one I offer my clients. I tell them, "Whenever your partner becomes defensive for no apparent reason, consider the possibility that you have become accusing without realizing it."

I hold myself responsible for a client's defensiveness in the same way that a diamond cutter holds himself or herself responsible for making a faulty cut and shattering the diamond. The diamond cutter's mistake is tapping the diamond at the wrong spot. My mistake is directing attention to the wrong issue or even entering on the side of the harsh internal taskmaster. When Carl Rogers and Heinz Kohut talked about maintaining an empathic stance, they meant, among other things, intervening at the right spot—as did Otto Fenichel (1941) when he talked about making surface rather than deep interpretations.

The therapist's task is in some ways more difficult than the diamond cutter's. Whereas the diamond cutter can puzzle over a gem for months before making a single tap, the therapist often has only a few seconds before he or she must make an intervention (or decide not to make one). In the course of a 50-minute session, the therapist may make a great many interventions. So the therapist is going to make mistakes. For me, making mistakes means:

> Reinforcing the taskmaster's injunctions rather than providing a platform from which the client can look at them.
> Becoming accusing or defensive (shifting into an adversarial interaction with the client) without knowing it.

Therefore, I have tried to develop skill at noticing when I do these things and in dealing with the effects.

An Example of a Therapist's Becoming Accusing without Knowing It

Marie and Paul spend several minutes blaming each other for a problem. I suggest a "nonblaming" alternative:

> Paul, as you're saying, you see Marie as responsible for this problem. Marie, you see Paul as responsible. But there's another way of looking at the situation that blames no one. And this other way is that each of you was struggling with a difficult feeling. Marie, you were feeling alone, and, Paul, you were feeling—

I hope to intrigue Marie and Paul with this nonblaming way of looking at their situation. But Paul says:

> Yes, well, if that's what Marie was feeling, why didn't she come right out and tell me instead of attacking me?

I say to myself:

> Paul is arguing with me—which means that I may be arguing with him without knowing it and that we're now in an adversarial

interaction. If so, Paul probably won't listen to what I'm saying—
although, of course, from his point of view, I'm not listening to
him either. On the other hand, if I found just the right argument,
he *might* listen. I'll give it one more try.

In response to Paul's insistence that Marie should have said what
she said in a nicer way, I say:

> Well, by the time she told you, she had built up a lot of steam about
> it—and so when she opened her mouth to tell you, what came
> out was the steam.

But Paul says:

> Well, then, why didn't she tell me earlier, *before* she built up all that
> steam?

I say to myself:

> Well, *that* apparently wasn't the right argument, since Paul instinc-
> tively rebutted it. I'm beginning to think that maybe there *isn't* a
> "right argument"—that we're in an adversarial interaction, and that
> Paul isn't going to listen to anything I say. And maybe also, I'm
> not really listening to him.

Looking back on the conversation between Paul and me, I try to
figure out how we have gotten into this adversarial interaction. I say to
myself:

> Maybe it happened a couple of exchanges back, when I said, "Paul,
> as you're saying, you see Marie as responsible for the problem.
> . . . But there's another way of looking at the situation that
> blames no one." Paul might have felt I was blaming *him* for blam-
> ing Marie. And, now that I think about it, that's what I was do-
> ing, along with blaming Marie for blaming Paul. And he might
> have taken *further* offense just a little later when I told him: "Well,
> by the time she told you, she had built up a lot of steam about
> it—and so when she opened her mouth to tell you, what came
> out was the steam."

> What I *thought* I was saying was this: "Paul, yes, sure, you're under-
> standably not going to like being yelled at. And you're understand-

ably going to want to yell back or object in some other way. But I want you to have the advantage of knowing that much of the bite of Marie's comment came from her having held it back."

What Paul probably heard (through the mediating voice of his harsh inner taskmaster) was this: "Stupid, can't you see that Marie was holding her feelings back—that's why they came out so explosively. You shouldn't take it so personally. You're oversensitive. Furthermore, why do you think she was holding her feelings back? It's because you always take things so personally."

Hearing it through this voice, Paul became defensive. He said, appealing to Response 20, "Well, why didn't she tell me earlier, *before* she built up all that steam?"

I provoked Paul's internal recriminations—I took the taskmaster's side. Furthermore, I failed to take into account Paul's "feeling-angry-at-Marie, wanting-to-make-sure-she-is-properly-reproached-for-what-I-feel-she-has-been-doing" state of mind. Here is what I might have said if I had taken it into account:

Well, maybe you feel that I'm letting Marie off too easily—that I'm excusing her. Maybe you feel that, despite what I'm saying, in an important way Marie *is* to blame—that she ought to 'fess up to it, take responsibility for it, and be held accountable for it. Maybe you feel that she doesn't appreciate how affected you are by what she says, and that I don't either.

Every day in my work with couples—in fact, every hour—I see partners attempt to have a conversation but, without knowing it, slip into adversarial interactions in which neither listens to the other. Instead, each tries to convince the other of his or her own point. Partners can look pretty ridiculous shifting back and forth between conversation and argument. I stopped thinking of them as ridiculous, however, when I realized that I was doing the same thing, not only with *my* own partner, but also with my clients. It is easy to feel mildly provoked and, without knowing it, snap into a "slightly-adversarial, slightly-argumentative, slightly-polarized" couple state or therapist–client interaction. It is easy to convince myself that I am in a conversation when I am really in an argument—as in the example I have just described, when I ignored the evidence that Paul and I were in an argument and gave it one more try.

What do I do when I conclude that I am in an adversarial interaction with a client?

I immediately take the client's side. As noted above, for instance, I could say to Paul, "Well, maybe you feel I'm letting Marie off too easily . . ."

And/or I create a platform from which I can confide in my clients about my arguing with them. For example, I could tell Paul, "It looks like I've been arguing with you about this."

Of course, once I am on a joint platform with Paul—that is, once I am talking nonargumentatively with him about my arguing—I am no longer arguing:

I've been so busy arguing—trying to convince you of my point—that I haven't been listening to your point. So let me listen. And, if I think back on what you were saying and trying to get me to see, I'd realize that it was that _____.

Creating a joint platform from which Paul and I can look at my arguing does not mean that I necessarily have to give up trying to make my point. In fact, I am now in a better position to make it:

In that argument we were having a moment ago, I wasn't able to convince you that _____. But I just thought of a better way to make my point—so I'd like to tell you about it and see if you find it convincing.

Instead of just trying to convince Paul of something, I am now telling him of my wish to convince him. By talking in a nonarguing way about our argument, I am inviting him onto the platform with me. And since I am no longer in an adversarial interaction with him, he may now be able to join me there, where he can listen to me—and I to him. If a joint platform is what is needed to get a couple relationship working well, then a joint platform is what is needed to get a *therapy* relationship working well.

Evenhandedness in Dealing with Partners

Like practically all other couples therapists, I try to avoid taking sides. And like practically all other couples therapists, I sometimes do it anyway—despite all my efforts.

So I try to become increasingly skillful at noticing when I've lost my evenhandedness, and in dealing with it when I do. One way to deal with it is behaviorally—that is, by immediately and temporarily taking the side of the partner whose position I may have been neglecting. Another way—my preferred way—is to establish a joint platform from which to talk with partners about my lack of evenhandedness. For example:

THERAPIST: Marie, I've just realized that we've spent a lot of time developing Paul's point of view, so I'm wondering whether you feel that I'm siding with Paul and that no one is interested in *your* point of view.
MARIE: Well, actually, I *was* starting to worry about getting my chance.

Of course, in acknowledging that I have not been looking at things from Marie's point of view, I *am* looking at things from her point of view. She goes on:

I don't think the two of you understand what it's like to be a working mother with no time for herself. (*To Paul*) I know you help a lot with the kids, the housework, and everything else, but it's still up to me to organize things and make sure everything gets done.

I try to create a platform from which the three of us can look at Marie's feeling that Paul and I do not understand her. I focus our attention on this issue, and, in subsequent sessions, I refer back to it. For example, in the middle of the next session, I may say to Marie:

THERAPIST: Remember last time when you said you felt Paul and I weren't understanding—that neither of us appreciate what it's like to be a working mother. I wonder if you're feeling a bit of that now.
MARIE: Well, as a matter of fact—thanks for asking—yes, I *am*.

Marie can deal *behaviorally* with her feeling that I am not understanding: She can insist to Paul that they transfer to a female therapist, who she thinks might be more likely to understand. Or she can deal with her feeling *nonbehaviorally*, by creating a platform from which the three of us can talk about her feeling that I was not understanding. And, of course, she can do both: She can create a platform and, at the same time, push for transfer to a female therapist.

A joint platform puts everyone in a better position. It certainly puts me in one. I can use the partners as resources to help me detect whether or not I am taking sides. I do not have to rely solely on my own judgment. Instead of always having to act in ways that make it clear I am being evenhanded, I now have some leeway. When, as inevitably happens, I depart from neutrality, I have a way to deal with it: I can talk with them. And since I am able to talk with the partners about it, it becomes easier temporarily and purposely to *take* sides. I can say to Paul:

> I'm going to take Marie's side for a moment and see if I can convince you that, in a way that you're not realizing, maybe you're *not* understanding how she feels.

And/or I can say to Marie:

> I'm going to take Paul's side now just to see if I can convince you that he *might* be appreciating more about how you're feeling than you think.

By making it explicit that I am taking sides, I can do so without the usual negative effects—without leading Paul (or Marie) to wonder:

> Is it my imagination, or is Wile taking Marie's (Paul's) side?
> If it *is* my imagination, does it mean that I'm being oversensitive?
> If it *isn't* my imagination, what does *that* mean?
> Does it mean that I'm wrong and Marie (Paul) is right?
> Does it mean that Wile likes Marie (Paul) more than he does me?
> Does it mean that I'm unlikable?
> Does it mean that Wile is unfair?
> Does it mean that he favors women (men)?
> Do I have the right to complain?

Feelings of this sort and other sorts occur throughout therapy—and throughout life. My goal is to increase partners' abilities to confide in each other about them. The problem is not these troubling feelings in themselves, but rather the absence of a platform from which to look at them and to put them in perspective.

Without such a platform, these troubling feelings will get consigned to the collection of unintegrated, unresolved, and unspoken feelings that we amass throughout our lives. Ultimately, that is the value of the platform: to rescue our feelings from this heap.

Establishing a platform is my major way to:

> Help clients deal with the problems that arise in their lives and in their relationships.
> Help me deal with the problems that arise in my life and in my relationships.
> Help clients rescue their feelings from the heap of unintegrated, unresolved, and unspoken feelings that they amass throughout their lives.

Help me rescue my feelings from the heap of unintegrated, unresolved, and unspoken feelings that I amass throughout my life.

Help clients deal with problems that arise in their relationship
with me.

Help me deal with problems that arise in my therapeutic work (my
relationship) with them.

Help me recognize and deal with my unknowingly shifting into an
adversarial interaction with clients.

Help me deal with my nonevenhandedness in my work with
couples.

RECOVERING FROM THE FIGHT

Since fights are unavoidable, I place my emphasis on improving the couple's ability to recover from them.

CHAPTER 17

First Attempts
at a Recovery Conversation

After imagining the couples therapy session that Marie and Paul might have if they were to come to see me the day after the fight, let us return to the evening of the fight and see how they try to recover from it themselves.

And let us give them the advantage of having just read this book. In fact, let us imagine how the fight might go if Marie and Paul were to have mastered everything in this book so far. When Marie storms into the living room and says, "You never talk to me any more," Paul, calling upon his expertise, would remember—

Nothing. He would snap into the "defensive" state of mind, which means forgetting everything in the book that cannot be incorporated into one of the 44 defensive responses. If he were to use the book at all, it would be as a weapon in his defense. For instance:

> You apparently didn't learn anything from Wile's book. You're not going to get anywhere by jumping down my throat. Go read the book again.

Only later, when Paul no longer feels accused and is thus no longer in the "defensive" state of mind, might he be able to use the book in a way that is not just part of the fight—or even to remember what is in the book.

But when is "later"? Pretty soon—because the fight has cleared the air for him. It has given him the chance to voice feelings that he was suffering in silence. He has called Marie a nag—and he feels better for it. He is ready to make peace.

Marie is *not* ready. She has been *called* a nag. Rather than clearing the air for her, the fight has dirtied it. It has left her with even *more* feelings to suffer in silence. While Paul walks around the block recuperating in the rain, she is in the kitchen fuming.

Peacemaking

By the time Paul gets back to the house, his anger has subsided. He has shifted from the "hating-Marie" state of mind to the "feeling-better-about-her, distressed-by-the-tension-and-anger, wanting-to-make-peace" state of mind. He considers the following peacemaking plans:

1. Offering to help with dinner.
2. Giving Marie what she says she wants: more talking.
3. Putting my arms around her.
4. Trying to make up by having sex.
5. Joking around.
6. Admitting it was my fault.
7. Apologizing.
8. Promising to change.
9. Trying to talk it out. And, if necessary:
10. Following Marie from room to room in an effort to try to talk it out.
11. Waiting until Marie cools down—and then trying any of the above.
12. Leaving it to Marie to make the first move.
13. Going on as if nothing has happened and hoping that Marie will do the same.

Here is how Paul sorts through these possibilities:

Possible Plan	*Paul's Evaluation*
1. Offering to help with dinner.	But Marie might still be fuming, in which case she'd probably say something like, "Leave me alone and get out of the kitchen! And I don't even understand why you're in here? Isn't some foreign-language channel still doing the News?"
2. Giving Marie what she says she wants: more talking. I could say, "Tell me what happened to you today."	But she might say, "I'll tell you what happened. I came home from a hard day at work and got called a nag. Anything else you want to know about my day?"

3. Putting my arms around her. I could go over to her and give her a hug.

But that's not my style. Also, she might pull away—and I'd feel like a fool.

4. Trying to make up by having sex. I could give her an *extra long* hug showing her that I'm interested in having sex tonight.

That *is* my style—sex is how I try to make things better. Unfortunately, things have to be better first before Marie is ever interested in sex.

5. Joking around. I could say, "Next time let's fight when it isn't raining; I got soaked."

But she could say, "Anyone who hits and runs deserves what he gets."

6. Admitting it was my fault. I could say, "I had a bad day at work and I took it out on you."

But Marie could say, "I'm *tired* of your taking things out on me."

7. Apologizing. I could say, "I'm sorry I called you a nag."

But Marie could say, "Apologies are cheap. I don't want apologies, I want change."

8. Promising to change. So maybe I should just *start* with "I promise never to call you names again."

But Marie could say, "I'll believe it when I see it."

9. Trying to talk it out. What I *should* do, of course—what most books say you should do—is go to Marie and tell her, "We need to talk."

She'd never expect to hear that from me. I'd have to pick her up off the floor. And then, once she had her wits back, she'd probably say, "Talk? Sure. We need to talk about how you avoid me, how you call me names, how you . . ."

10. Following Marie from room to room in an effort to talk it out. I know what *Marie* would do if she were in my position. She'd follow me wherever I went insisting that we talk it out. In fact, I wonder why she isn't doing that now.

But I'm *glad* she isn't. It always makes things worse.

11. Waiting until Marie cools down and then trying any of the above. Since Marie is going to reject *anything* I say, maybe I should just wait until she cools down.

Yes, I like that one.

12. Leaving it to *Marie* to make the first move. She's the one who's being difficult; why should I have to reach out to her?

But she'd just use it against me later. She'd say, "I'm tired of always being the one who holds out the olive branch."

13. Going on as if nothing has happened. I could go into the kitchen and ask, "What's for dinner?" Of course, it's risky to be so casual this soon after the fight. She might give me the silent treatment, and I'd feel like I blew it. What I think I'll do is keep a low profile the rest of the evening and then wake up tomorrow as if nothing's happened.

I know that's not the best thing to do—you're supposed to talk things out. But it's the only plan that's ever worked for me.

So Paul ends up doing what he usually does—going on as if the fight never occurred.

And he may be wise to do so. True, what he *thinks* he should do—talk about the fight—has an important advantage: It can lead to a mutual understanding about what caused the fight. But, of course, that is not what *usually* happens. What usually happens when partners try to talk about a fight is that they simply rekindle it.

If Paul is going to have any interest at all in talking to Marie, he will need to feel that there is at least a chance that re-airing the fight will not simply cause it to flare up again. So I am going to present seven principles that give him that chance. The first five are discussed below; the sixth and seventh are discussed in Chapter 18.

Principles for Talking about a Fight

It is several hours later. After ignoring Paul at dinner, Marie disappears to read to Billy. Paul feels abandoned. Later, after they put the kids to bed, Paul overhears Marie telling her friend Nancy on the phone, "Paul's been a real jerk tonight." Although Paul doesn't like Marie's talking about him like this, he is somewhat heartened by her tone. There is something almost cheerful in it, as if she is no longer angry at him. And there are worse things than being called a jerk.

Since Marie seems to be coming around, Paul snaps into the "feeling-more-hopeful, maybe-this-evening-can-be-rescued-after-all" state. So he looks up what the Wile book recommends doing after a fight. And he reads:

> Recovery conversations: There are always going to be fights. You cannot avoid them entirely. What you can do, however, is to become skillful at recovering from them by learning how to talk about them afterwards.

If Paul is going to try to have a recovery conversation—that is, if he is going to try to talk about this fight—now is the time, since Marie seems to be feeling better toward him. Of course, that is not what Paul's instincts tell him to do. They tell him—they *scream* at him—"Marie is feeling better about you. Why press your luck? If it ain't broke, don't fix it."

Having just read the book, Paul is intrigued by the possibility of trying to have a recovery conversation. Overriding his instincts, he decides to give it a try. He begins by mentally reviewing the fight: how Marie came into the TV room and said, "You never talk to me any more"; how he tried to explain himself but she refused to listen; and how, in frustration, he called her a nag.

Marie is in the bedroom reading. Paul walks in, clears his throat, takes a deep breath, and—what?

He is about to say, "You always choose the moment I sit down to relax to pick a fight." But he remembers:

• **Principle 1: "I statements" versus "you statements."** "You statements" (e.g., "You always _____") are likely to rekindle the fight. "I statements" (e.g., "I feel hurt when you _____") give you at least a chance of not rekindling it.

Every book Paul has ever read about relationships tells him that he should avoid making "you statements"—and here, in his very first comment, he is about to make one. His "You always choose the moment I sit down to relax to pick a fight" is a clear "you statement."

Of course, the comment that began the fight—Marie's "You never talk to me any more"—was itself a "you statement." The evening would have gone differently if, instead, Marie had said something like "*I miss* our not talking the way we used to." Paul would probably have taken that as a friendly overture rather than as an attack.

Of course, Paul is in no position to complain about Marie's "you statements," since he made several of his own:

You can't expect just one person to satisfy all your needs.
Why can't you appreciate the good things we have instead of always dwelling on the bad?
You worry about things too much and let them bother you more than you should.
I'd give you a little human treatment if you weren't such a nag.

The problem with "you statements"—the reason they fuel a fight—is that they are attacks, and the other person doesn't feel like doing anything except defending or attacking back. Paul's, "You always choose the moment I sit down to relax to pick a fight" would snap Marie into a "needing-to-defend-myself, wanting-to-attack-back" state of mind. It would temporarily eliminate Marie's wish, even her ability, to express her feelings—that is, to make "I statements." Marie would no longer know, or even care, what her feelings are. Her attention would be focused entirely on defending and retaliating.

The problem with "you statements," in other words, is that they make it difficult for the other person to make "I statements."

Paul's success in applying the principles in the book—his sense of satisfaction in being able to remember the "'I-statements'-versus-'you-statements'" principle—snaps him into a state of mind in which he now feels like making an "I statement." So he interrupts the "you statement" he has just begun and replaces it with an "I statement":

> You always choose just the moment . . . I mean, when you came in and said, "You never talk to me any more," I felt blindsided. I saw the first chance I had all day to relax going up in smoke.

Paul hopes his "I statement" will bring Marie around. He is disappointed, therefore, when Marie sits there glum-faced. But then he remembers:

• **Principle 2: Taking your partner's point of view.** "I statements" are efforts to get your partner to appreciate your point of view. You are saying, "I feel this" or "I feel that." But such efforts often lead your partner to feel that you do not appreciate *his* or *her* point of view. In other words, "I statements" aren't enough. Your partner needs to feel that you appreciate his or her point of view before he or she will be able to appreciate yours.

In saying, "I saw the first chance I had all day to relax going up in smoke," Paul is doing what people typically do when they try to talk about a fight: repeating points made during the fight (or presenting new ones). He feels that if only he were able to make the right points—or say them often enough or with sufficient emphasis—Marie would understand. He does not realize that what Marie needs at the moment is for him to appreciate the points that *she* has been trying to make.

And there is another problem. Everyone knows that putting an "I feel" at the beginning of a sentence does not guarantee an "I statement"—as in "I feel you are a jerk." Less well known is that even *true* "I statements" often contain implied "you statements":

Paul is expressing his feelings—he is making an "I statement"—when he says "I felt blindsided. I saw the first chance I had all day to relax going up in smoke."

But it would be hard for anyone in Marie's position not to hear Paul's comment, at least in part, as a "you statement"—that is, as "*You* blindsided me, and *you* interfered with the first chance I had all day to relax."

Even if Paul's "I statement" did not contain a hidden "you statement," Marie might still not want to hear it. She needs him to appreciate how she feels before she will able to appreciate how he feels.

In fact, as I have emphasized in Chapter 14, that is what a couple fight is: a deadlock in which one partner's feeling that his or her own point is not being appreciated makes it impossible to appreciate the other's point. Paul and Marie's fight exemplifies this:

During the fight, Paul had no interest whatsoever in considering Marie's point, which was that he had not been talking much to her recently, until she acknowledged his point, which was that she was bringing it up in an angry and provocative way.

But Marie had no interest in considering Paul's point, which was that she was bringing up her point in an angry and provocative way, until Paul acknowledged her point, which was that Paul had not been talking much to her recently.

The way Paul could make it possible for Marie to appreciate his point is by appreciating hers. He could do this, among other ways, by saying:

I've been thinking more about what you said before. You're right, I haven't been talking much recently—and I hadn't realized it.

I finally realized what you were trying to tell me—I was so angry at the time that I couldn't hear it—and it's that . . .

You know, part of what made it so hard to hear—and why I got so upset—was my worry that you might be right and that I *hadn't* been talking to you much recently.

I can see why you might be unhappy with me tonight. There were important things to talk about, and I disappeared to watch the News.

Typically, Paul would have no wish to say *any* of these things, since, as I have said, he would need Marie to acknowledge his point before he would have any desire to acknowledge hers. But he is pleased by his ability to figure out what the deadlock is. And this satisfaction puts him in a state of mind in which he *is* prepared to try to appreciate her point, even though she has not first appreciated his. Having just told her, "I felt blindsided," he now adds:

> And what really bothered me—what upset me the most—is that I was afraid you might be right.

Paul has also told her, "I saw the first chance I had all day to relax going up in smoke." He now adds:

> Of course, given our schedules, maybe your only chance to talk to *me* went up in smoke when you saw me heading for the TV.

Paul has found two ways to look at things from Marie's point of view. And he hopes that this will bring her around. But again she just sits there staring into her magazine, which is more than he can take:

> This is hard. Give me a little help, will you? Don't just sit there like a bump on a log.

Having put his all into seeing things from Marie's point of view, Paul is unprepared to deal with her lack of response. He has forgotten:

• **Principle 3: Nice-guy backlash.** There is always the danger when you reach out to (or do something special for) your partner—even without the thought of reciprocation—that you'll suddenly resent its absence. You feel taken advantage of, taken for granted, out on a limb, or just plain foolish.

There is just so long that you can remain nonaccusing and nondefensive while your partner continues to be irritable and unresponsive, without losing patience and becoming irritable and unresponsive yourself. By the time your partner comes around and begins to respond positively, it is too late. You feel so out of sorts that you no longer care. You have snapped into "nice-guy backlash" (a term coined by a friend of mine, Patricia Blanche).

You and your partner may now change roles, with your partner trying to bring *you* around. The fight may continue for some time, with the two of you taking turns reaching out and then, when the other responds too slowly, lashing out.

Nice-guy backlash is unavoidable. There will always be moments when you find yourself resenting your partner's not responding or not reciprocating. Instead of trying to avoid nice-guy backlash, I recommend developing skill in recognizing it and recovering from it. Here is what Paul might say to Marie if he already had these skills:

> Here I am beating you over the head for not coming around immediately. Just because I *want* you to stop being mad doesn't mean that you should *have* to. Maybe you're not ready. Or maybe I'm not doing a good enough job bringing you around.

This statement would be likely to soften the impact of Paul's nice-guy backlash. Unfortunately, Paul lacks the skills to recognize and recover from nice-guy backlash, and is unable to make such a statement. And without it, the fight quickly escalates. Marie responds to Paul's provocative "Give me a little help, will you? Don't just sit there like a bump on a log" with this:

> I didn't ask you to come in here.

Paul can't stand it. Marie is turning his effort to talk about the fight—that is, to try to make things better—into a weapon against him. He wishes he had followed his instincts and kept his mouth shut. He feels like putting my book on a low shelf where the cat can get at it.

And here is why it is difficult to have a successful recovery conversation: There are traps everywhere. And there is very little margin for error:

> Paul starts out well: He remembers Principle 1 ("I statements").
> And he remembers Principle 2 ("taking your partner's point of view").
> But he forgets Principle 3 ("nice-guy backlash"), and the result is an immediate rekindling of the fight.

But there is a way out. Paul can deal with forgetting Principle 3 by remembering:

• **Principle 4: *Expecting* to rekindle the fight.** Since it is impossible to avoid rekindling the fight, expect it and plan for it.

Marie and Paul are watching each other like hawks. She is all set to see him as blaming her for being accusing—which, of course, is what he has been doing. And Paul is all set to see her as blaming him for being defensive—as *she* has been doing. No matter how hard they try, one or the other of them will inevitably say something that the other will interpret as accusing or defensive. The result will be a rekindling of the fight. So I recommend:

> Expecting such rekindling—that is, appreciating how easy it is to slip back into the fight—so you do not become so discouraged when you do.
> Developing skill in noticing and recovering from this rekindling.

A major element in having recovery conversations is learning how to make on-the-spot recoveries when the conversation itself turns sour, and, if you cannot, remembering that rekindling is bound to happen. Paul would be making such an on-the-spot recovery if he were to respond to Marie's "I didn't ask you to come in here" with this:

> Hey, you're not supposed to say that. You're supposed to say, "I'm *glad* you came in here." Of course, I can't expect you to be glad to see me if I'm going to accuse you of sitting there like a bump on a log.

Such a statement is likely to soften the effect of his nice-guy back-lash; that is, it is likely to enable him to make a recovery from the just-being-rekindled fight. Unfortunately, like most of us, Paul is not skill-ful in making such recoveries. Instead, he deals with Marie's swipe at him ("I didn't ask you to come in here") by swiping back:

PAUL: Well, I had to come in here. Otherwise you'd spend all night here alone, sulking like a 2-year-old.
MARIE (*defending herself*): I wasn't sulking. I was reading. Anyway, why would you even care? You just see me as a nag.

Immediately Paul snaps into the "feeling-stung, all-I-can-think-of-is-how-to-sting-back, defensive, losing-my-ability-to-think" state of mind—which is too bad, because Marie has just said something impor-tant. She is finally telling him why she has been unresponsive up to this point: She is still fuming over being called a nag. She needs to tell him how upset she feels before she can make peace.

So it is a breakthrough: Marie is finally saying what she needs to say to be able to listen to what Paul wants to say.

Paul does not see it as a breakthrough, of course. It's hard to see that Marie is saying something that is going to lead to peace, when at the moment she just seems to be getting more upset. If Paul is to recog-nize that she is saying is a step toward making things better, he needs to know:

• **Principle 5: Looking for the missing piece.** If your partner is not listening to you, something is probably stuck in his or her craw; that is, there is something he or she needs to figure out and get across before being able to listen to you. Similarly, if *you* are not listening to your partner, there is probably something you need to figure out and say.

If Paul were to recognize Marie's "You just see me as a nag" as the missing piece—as what she needs to say in order to be able to listen to him—he might take heart. He might be glad that she is finally getting it out.

But he does not recognize it as such. And he feels too upset about having called Marie a nag—he knows how much it hurts her—to be able to tolerate her complaint about it. It's ironic. If Paul didn't feel it was so unforgivable to call Marie a nag, he wouldn't be so upset about her being sore about it. The minute she reminds him of what he said, he lashes out defensively:

PAUL: Look, I'm trying to work things out between us. Can't you appreciate that? Why do you have to make things even harder than they already are?

MARIE: I'm not making things harder. It's *you* who messed everything up by calling me a nag.

PAUL: But you should be over it by now. You should be like me: get angry, get it out, and forgive and forget.

MARIE: Easy for you to say. You wouldn't "forgive and forget" so quickly if someone called *you* a name you despised.

Paul needs Marie to be over it by now (or, preferably, not to have become upset about it in the first place) because he feels so bad about calling her a nag. He tells Marie that she should forgive and forget. He doesn't recognize that her effort to talk about it now is her *way* to forgive and forget.

So, while Marie is telling him something ("You just see me as a nag") that, if he could tolerate it, might enable her to listen to him, he is hearing this very same statement as something that makes him completely unable to listen to her. He sputters—

This is getting nowhere.

—and rushes out of the bedroom.

Back in the TV room, feeling frustrated, Paul wonders what happened.

Skeptic: I'll tell you what happened. This proves exactly what I've been saying all along: It's crazy to try to talk about your fights. Look how hard Paul tried—even using all your fancy principles—and the conversation *still* didn't work out.

Wile: Yes, but . . .

Skeptic: Look, *here's* what Paul should have done. He should have said, "Listen, Marie. I'm sorry I called you a nag. I didn't really mean it."

Wile: Well sure. Apologizing can help—sometimes. If Paul were to say that, Marie might see that he *does* realize that she was hurt. On the other hand, Marie might take his apology as his simply trying to get her off his back.

Skeptic: But she could also be *touched* by it—particularly if Paul is a person who rarely apologizes.

Wile: Well, sure . . .

Skeptic: But wait—I didn't finish. Paul should say, "I'm sorry." And *then*—and here's the important part—he should keep his mouth shut. Because it's trying to talk about the fight that's causing the problem. And then Marie should say, "That's okay; forget about it"—and then she should keep *her* mouth shut. They should kiss and make up. Because that's the beauty of an apology: It can end the fight without anyone having to discuss anything. In fact, it'd be a good idea if Marie and Paul were to make love or watch television so they *can't* talk about the fight.

Wile: That's a terrific Hollywood ending, but if Marie and Paul don't talk about their fights, how are they going to learn anything from them? There's important information about a relationship hidden in a fight, but it takes a bit of talking to dig it out.

Skeptic: That sounds good in theory, but I'd forget about "learning something from a fight." We're talking about keeping it from getting out of hand and destroying the relationship.

Wile: Well, I think there's a way that Marie and Paul can learn something from the fight and still get to keep their relationship. And, remember, I've described only *five* of the seven principles. The last two may provide the needed edge.

CHAPTER 18

The "Admitting–Admitting" Couple State

Paul is back in the TV room, feeling frustrated. He has the following internal conversation:

I hate it when Marie holds a grudge.

Why can't she let things roll off her back like I do?

Okay, I called her a nag. Why is that so horrible? No one ever keeled over and died at the sound of the word.

And she *was* kind of a nag. She should be honest enough to admit it.

I hadn't even gotten my coat off, for heaven's sake, and she was in my face with a list of everything that went wrong today.

And then I'm sitting there watching the News and she storms in like an invading army and attacks me for not talking enough.

If that's not nagging, what is?

Okay, so calling her a nag wasn't the smartest thing I ever did.

In fact, it was pretty stupid. It's the kind of thing Dad would say to Mom. I can't stand the thought that I'm getting to be like him.

Of course, I'm not *entirely* like him. I help with the kids—and with everything else. Dad didn't even know where the food was kept.

In fact, I'm hardly like him at all. He didn't talk to us kids except to discipline us, and he never played with me at all. And I have a great relationship with Jeannie and Billy.

Marie should be grateful she's married to me.

Hey look, I'm not perfect. I say some harsh things sometimes. Everyone does—even *Marie*.

What was it she called me last week when I came home a little late from basketball? "Irresponsible."

Where does she get off calling me that?

Of course, where do *I* get off calling her a nag?

If she's reacting to my calling her a nag the way I reacted to her calling me irresponsible, then she must be pretty upset.

Maybe that's why she just sat there saying nothing when I tried to talk with her.

In the course of this conversation with himself, Paul has shifted from accusing Marie to sympathizing with her. How has that happened?

With Marie no longer there to interrupt him, Paul has a chance to make his case, at least to himself: "She *was* kind of a nag. She should be honest enough to admit it. I hadn't even gotten my coat off, for heaven's sake, and she was in my face with a list of everything that went wrong today."

Paul gets enough satisfaction out of establishing Marie's contribution to the problem—taking the blame off himself by putting it on her—that he is then prepared to consider *his* contribution: "Okay, so calling her a nag wasn't the smartest thing I ever did. In fact, it was pretty stupid. It's the kind of thing Dad would say to Mom. I can't stand the thought that I'm getting to be like him."

Bringing in his concern about being like his father allows him to confront it: "Of course, I'm not *entirely* like him. . . . In fact, I'm not like him at all. . . . Marie should be grateful she's married to me."

Viewing himself in this more positive light, Paul is then able to tolerate his imperfections—that is, he is able to see them as human rather than fatal: "Hey look, I'm not perfect. I say some harsh things sometimes. Everyone does—even *Marie*."

And, remembering how he felt when Marie called him "irresponsible," Paul is then able to appreciate how Marie probably felt when he called her a nag: "If she's reacting to my calling her a nag the way I reacted to her calling me irresponsible, then she must be pretty upset. Maybe that's why she just sat there saying nothing when I tried to talk with her."

In short, how does Paul switch from blaming Marie to sympathizing with her?

He needs to establish her contribution to the problem before he can look at his; he needs to get on his own side before he can get on hers.

And he needs to remember how he felt when she called him "irresponsible" to realize how she must have felt when he called her a nag.

So, just thinking about the situation without Marie around has put Paul in a better state of mind. He is on the platform. That is, he is thinking about his fight with Marie in a nonaccusing and nondefensive way. And it has enabled him finally to see what is bugging Marie: his calling her a nag. He has found the missing piece.

The "missing-piece" principle—Principle 5 (which I have described in the preceding chapter)—is crucial. Once Paul has the idea that there *is* a missing piece—that is, that there is a point that, if Marie can get it established, will enable her to listen to him—Paul will be in a position to look for it.

Of course, in order to be interested in finding the missing piece for Marie, Paul needs, as a first step, to find the missing piece for himself:

• **Principle 6:** *Two* **conflicting missing pieces.** At any moment in a fight, *each* partner has something sticking in his or her craw; that is, each partner has something he or she needs to be able to get the other to hear before being able to listen to anything from the other. Unfortunately, what each partner says in the effort to get the other to listen typically leaves the other feeling *un*listened to.

Paul needs to know that Marie is suffering from not having gotten her point across—and that he is too:

Before she can listen to anything Paul has to say, Marie needs him to appreciate that his calling her a nag was hurtful.
But before he can listen to anything Marie has to say, Paul needs her to see that his calling her a nag was not so terrible.

What is needed is for someone to go first:

If Paul were to go first—if he were to say, "As soon as I used the word 'nag' I knew I'd gone over the line and really hurt you"—then Marie might begin to be able to listen to him.

If Marie were to go first and say, "I know that in the heat of battle people sometimes call each other some pretty awful things; you called me a nag, and I called you a few names as well"—Paul might now begin to be able to listen to her.

Unfortunately, neither can go first. Marie needs Paul to acknowledge that what he said was hurtful before she will be able to forgive him for it. But Paul needs her to forgive him for it before he will be able to acknowledge that he said something hurtful. This is what a couple fight is: a stalemate in which what each says in the effort to make his or her point just leads the other to feel that his or her own point is being ignored.

> In Paul's effort to get Marie to acknowledge that his calling her a nag was not so awful and unforgivable, Paul says, "Why do you have to make things even harder than they already are? . . . You should be like me: get angry, get it out, and forgive and forget." But that just leads Marie to feel that Paul doesn't appreciate how badly his calling her a nag hurt her.
> In her effort to get Paul to appreciate that his calling her a nag was hurtful, Marie says, "You wouldn't 'forgive and forget' so quickly if someone called *you* a name you despised." But that just leads Paul to feel that Marie sees his calling her a nag as unforgivable.

So Marie and Paul are stuck. The "two-conflicting-missing-pieces" principle (Principle 6) shows why they are stuck.

But how is that a help?

Well, it was not much of a help during the fight, when they were in such "frustrated, narrowed-down, unable-to-listen, unable-to-think" states of mind that they couldn't even remember Principle 6. During fights, people do not care about Principle 6—or about any of the other principles.

So it is only *after* the fight and, in fact, in his second attempt to make up, when Paul feels less angry and is able to think again—when he is sufficiently able to take his own side that he can now take Marie's—that he is able to remember Principle 6. He says to himself:

> Wile says that when partners are in a fight, what each says in the effort to be heard just leads the other to feel unheard.

Which is all the reminder Paul needs to begin to wonder: "What was the point that Marie was trying to make that was driving her crazy and getting her more and more upset because she couldn't make it? And what was the point that *I* couldn't make?" He concludes:

> Well, it's obvious. Marie needed me to see that calling her a nag was hurtful. And I needed her to tell me that my calling her a nag wasn't so hurtful. No wonder we got so stuck.

Inspired by this discovery, Paul marches back into the bedroom and tells Marie:

> When I called you a nag earlier tonight, I knew I had done something really stupid. That's why I had to get out of the house so fast—because I knew I had blown it big time.

Immediately Marie's body relaxes, which indicates to Paul that he is on the right track; his calling her a nag *is* what was sticking in her craw. Marie is not fully satisfied, however:

> Well, why did you say it then?

Marie has taken advantage of Paul's admission to grind his face in it, which upsets Paul. He is about to succumb to nice-guy backlash. But he thinks he sees a general relaxing in her and a softening in her tone and that enables him to hang on. Marie continues:

> You completely ruined the evening.

He has only been hanging by a thread, and this pushes him over the edge:

> *You're* the one who ruined the evening—you *were* nagging me.

And now the gloves are off.

MARIE: I knew it! That's what you really think, down deep.
PAUL: Yes. I do. You're just like my mother.

Somewhere within Paul a voice is screaming at him: "What are you saying? Put a lid on it. You're running amok and you'll regret it—you're *already* regretting it."

MARIE: See, *that's* the problem: You see me as your mother. We're not going to get anywhere as long as you keep thinking I'm your mother the nag.
PAUL: Leave my mother out of it, will you?
MARIE: *You* brought her into it. You said I was just like her.
PAUL: Well, you *are*. You said I don't talk enough? That's what my mother always told my father. She'd say, "Turn off the TV, George, and talk to me."
MARIE: Oh, so *that's* where you learned it.

PAUL: Learned *what*?

MARIE: How to hide out in front of the TV. You got it from your father.

PAUL (*icily*): I would very much appreciate your leaving my father out of this. First you bring in my mother and now it's my father. Is there anyone else in my family you want to enlist in this war?

MARIE: *You* were the one who brought them in, not me.

PAUL: I did *not*.

MARIE: Yes, you did. I remember distinctly.

PAUL: No, I didn't. *I* remember distinctly.

MARIE: I wish I'd taped it, so I could play it back at you.

Paul is growing weary of this fight. So he tries to think of a way to end it that will not leave him exposed if Marie again rebuffs him. Hoping for the best, he tries a joke:

If we did have a tape, Billy would probably find it and play it for the family at Thanksgiving.

By making a joke about the fight, Paul is offering Marie a way out of it. And she takes it; she, too, is weary. She smiles and says:

Your mom and dad would be horrified—they *never* fight.

Suddenly, Marie and Paul are in the "we're-in-it-together, we're-on-the-same-side, it's-us-against-them" couple state. Paul smiles back.

I'd love to see their reaction when they realize they're our model of how we don't want to be.

Marie's willingness to go along with Paul's joke—to join him in the "we're-in-it-together, we're-on-the-same-side, it's-us-against-them" couple state—emboldens him to say:

PAUL: How did we get into this fight, anyway?

MARIE: I don't know, but I sure wish we could get out of it.

Marie's "I wish we could get out of it" *is*, of course, already a way out of it. She is talking with Paul in a nonadversarial way about the adversarial interaction they have been having. After all his false starts, Paul has finally established a collaborative spirit, and they are now on the joint platform.

But what do they do now? Do they kiss and make up, forgive and forget, and say no more about it—as the Skeptic recommends? Or do they try to talk about it?

Ordinarily Paul would think it crazy to try to talk about the fight. But he remembers Principle 7 and is encouraged to give talking a chance. He hopes that Principle 7 will give them the edge they need to be able to talk about the fight without simply rekindling it.

• **Principle 7: Talking about only *your* contribution to the fight.** If you talk about your partner's contribution—saying, for example, "But it wasn't all me; you had a part in it too"—your partner is likely to feel, perhaps correctly, that you *mostly* blame him or her. If you talk exclusively about *your* contribution to the fight, however, your partner, grateful that you are acknowledging your role in the fight, is likely to begin to talk about his or hers.

Since Marie is all set to see Paul as blaming her—which, after all, is primarily what he has been doing—she needs clear, uninterrupted evidence that he is not. He cannot get away with the kind of half-discussion, half-blaming in which he (and nearly all partners) usually engage. If Paul is to avoid rekindling the fight, he can talk about his own contribution to it, but he cannot talk about Marie's. She will immediately assume that he mostly blames her. And she may be right.

At this early stage in the discussion, anything that hints of blaming—in fact, anything that is not clearly *non*blaming—can act as the starting bell for yet another round:

If Paul says, "We don't communicate well"—that is, if he attributes the problem to *both* of them—Marie may easily think that he really means *she* is the one who does not communicate well. And that *may* be what Paul means.

If Paul says, "I was wrong to call you a nag, but you were wrong to dump all your problems on me the minute I got home"—that is, if he talks about his contribution to the fight and then goes on to talk about hers—Marie may easily think that Paul's statement about his own contribution is just the preface and that his real message (what he really thinks—i.e., what comes after the "but") is that she is at fault. And she may be right.

If Paul says, "Well, okay, maybe it wasn't a good idea for me to leave in the middle of the fight, but I only did it to keep things from getting out of hand"—that is, if Paul tries to *justify* his behavior—Marie may easily think that he is denying responsibility. And, again, she may be right.

Actually, everyone already knows about Principle 7. That is, everyone knows that:

If you talk about your partner's contribution to the fight ("You yelled at me"), your partner is likely to talk about yours ("Well, that was only because you were sarcastic").

If you talk about *your* contribution to the fight, however, ("I feel bad that I got sarcastic"), your partner is likely to talk about his or her own contribution ("Well, I feel bad about yelling at you").

The value of Paul's admitting his contribution to the fight—the reason why it starts a discussion rather than another argument—is that it makes clear to Marie that he is neither blaming her nor denying responsibility.

Principle 7 may sound manipulative, like a "technique": Paul admits his role in the fight to soften Marie up and get her to admit hers. Fortunately—or unfortunately—Principle 7 is difficult to use as a "technique." Most people cannot carry it off. When they force themselves to speak only of their own contribution, they can only mumble a word or two before they begin to hint at their partners' contribution.

In order to stick with discussing his own contribution to the fight, Paul has to feel like it; he has to be in the right state of mind. And the way to be in the right state of mind is for Marie to stick to *her* contribution to the fight. In other words, if Paul is to feel like acknowledging his contribution to the fight, Marie will have to do so first. But if Marie is to feel like acknowledging her contribution to the fight, Paul will have to do so first. Someone has to go first. Or one of them has to ease into it.

Fortunately, Paul has already begun to ease into it. Marie's willingness to go along with his tension-reducing joke warms his heart. And her responding to his "How did we get into this fight, anyway?" by saying, "I don't know, but I sure wish we could get out of it," warms it a few degrees more. For the moment at least, Paul feels safe enough to make the following admission:

I know I said some pretty harsh things.

Paul is taking a chance. Marie could say, "You sure did! Maybe once in a while you should try thinking before you speak." And, immediately, Paul would be sorry he admitted anything. But, instead, Marie says:

Probably no worse than the things I said to you.

Paul's willingness to admit something has enabled Marie to admit something, which now enables Paul to admit something else:

I had a bad day at work, and I guess I took it out on you.

Is Paul pulling a number on Marie? Is he manipulatively talking about his part in the fight so that she will talk about hers?

No. He finds himself *wanting* to talk about his role in the fight. It takes no effort at all. He has snapped into an "appreciating-that-Marie-is-admitting-things, which-leads-me-to-feel-like-admitting-things" state of mind. And that snaps Marie into an "appreciating-that-Paul-is-admitting-things, which-leads-me-to-feel-like-admitting-things" state. At the moment, neither of them is even thinking about how the other might be at fault. Marie says:

> Well, it didn't help that I jumped on you with problems without giving you a chance to unwind first.

Just as Paul is talking about only his part in the fight, Marie is talking about only hers. And that is fortunate, because what each needs to continue to talk about only his or her part in the fight is for the other to continue to talk about only his or hers.

PAUL: I feel bad that I bailed out on you. There were clearly some important things you wanted to talk about.
MARIE: But I was wrong for laying them on you all at once.

A few minutes ago, Marie and Paul were caught up in an "attacking–defending" pattern. Now they are caught up in an "admitting–admitting" pattern.

The "admitting–admitting" pattern is delicately balanced. Any interruption—an accusing comment by either Marie or Paul, or simply something the other *hears* as accusing—can break the spell and throw the two of them back into the "attacking–defending" couple state. If Paul were to respond to Marie's "But I was wrong for laying [my problems] on you all at once" by saying, "Yes, well, you did come on pretty strong," that might break the unspoken agreement that each speak only of his or her own contribution to the fight. Marie might snap back, "Well, I had to come on strong to break through your thick skull"—and that would reignite the fight.

In order for this back-and-forth admitting to go on, each must also feel that the other is admitting enough in return. If Paul were to feel that Marie is not admitting her share, he would probably snap into nice-guy backlash and say something like "Of course, you had a part in it too"—which Marie is likely to hear as "In fact, you had the most important part." And that would also reignite the fight.

But, for the moment, each continues to feel that the other *is* admitting enough in return. In response to Marie's "But I was wrong for laying them on you all at once," Paul says:

Well, I can be pretty dense sometimes. Maybe you had to do it that way just to get my attention:

Paul is sympathizing with Marie for what she has to deal with in being married to him (his being "dense"). And in response, Marie sympathizes with him for what he has to deal with being married to her:

MARIE: But I didn't have to say it in such a pushy way. I know I can come on pretty strong—like when I came into the TV room and said, "You never talk to me any more." That was completely off the wall.
PAUL: But it *wasn't* completely off the wall. The worse things get at work, the more it seems I take it out on you. I *haven't* been talking much.

Amazing! Paul is saying spontaneously what Marie was working so hard earlier in the evening to get him to admit: that he has not been talking very much recently. And in response Marie makes an admission that is equally important to Paul:

Well, I know I get critical sometimes, so I can understand why you might be wary of talking to me.

Marie is hoping that Paul will not take advantage of her admission by telling her, "You can say that again." And her hope is answered. He says:

Well, you have reason to criticize. I know I haven't been the greatest company lately.

Paul is hoping that Marie will not take advantage of his admission to say, "You sure haven't." And she doesn't. Instead, she says:

Neither have I—I've been so caught up in work problems that I can't seem to leave them at work.

Marie is hoping that Paul will not take advantage of her admission by telling her, "You can say that again," or by giving her unwanted advice such as "Maybe you should quit your job." And he doesn't. Instead, he says:

It's been a hard time for both of us lately.

Each of them is counting on the other to abide by what I call the "talking-only-about-your-own-contribution-to-the-fight" principle—Principle 7.

In this way—by automatically, without even thinking about it, adhering to Principle 7—Marie and Paul have a conversation about the fight that does not simply rekindle it.

Skeptic: I must admit that you're starting to convince me. Maybe it *is* possible to talk about a fight without just rekindling it. I think I'll go home and try out Principle 7 with my husband. Heaven knows the timing would be right.

Wile: Well, actually, now I'm thinking that maybe *you're* right and it *isn't* possible.

Skeptic: Yes, but the very fact that you're saying that is a demonstration of one of your principles. I said that *you* might be right—and, in response, you said that *I* might be right.

Wile: And you *might* be. Look what it took! Paul had to keep persisting when his first attempts to talk about the fight didn't work out. Marie and Paul had to become weary of the fight at the *same moment*, so that when Paul tried to break the tension with a joke, Marie welcomed it. It took Marie's admitting enough in response to Paul's admitting things—and Paul's admitting enough in response to Marie's admitting things—to keep the "admitting–admitting" pattern going. At any moment, the whole structure could have come crashing down. I'm beginning to think that maybe you were right and that it might not be such a bad idea for Marie and Paul to just apologize and leave it at that.

Skeptic: You give up too easily. I'm still going to try it with my husband.

Wile: But listen—here's what I'm afraid will happen. You'll go home, make a stab at it, find it's harder than you bargained for, get discouraged, throw the book away, and forget the whole thing. Or, worse, you'll think that the book is okay, but that something's wrong with you or your husband, and *that's* why your attempt to talk didn't work out. That's the big problem we're all dealing with anyway—thinking there's something wrong with us or our partners or our relationships. I would hate for my book to contribute to that worry.

Skeptic: But what good are your principles if I don't try them? Why even bother to tell me about them?

Wile: Well, they're something to *know* rather than something to use.

Skeptic: But what's the point of knowing something if you don't use it? Do I just file all this away with what's left of my high school French?

Wile: Not exactly. And I'll tell you how it's different. Knowing these principles *is* using them. Let's say you know:

Principle 1: That your "you statements" are likely to rekindle the fight.

Principle 2: But that "I statements" aren't the whole answer either, since your husband needs you to appreciate his point of view (*his* "I statements") before he will be able to appreciate yours. (Not to mention the fact that your "I statements" are likely to contain hidden "you statements.")

Principle 3: That you're in constant danger of "nice-guy backlash," which can best be dealt with by expecting it and, though this might sound strange, planning for it.

Principle 4: That rekindling fights is inevitable and can best be dealt with by expecting and planning.

Principle 5: That if your husband isn't coming around, it's probably because there's something stuck in his craw that he needs to say.

Principle 6: That at any given moment in a fight, each of you has something stuck in his or her craw—and that is what maintains the fight.

Principle 7: That talking about your husband's contributions to the fight will rekindle it, but that talking about your own contributions won't rekindle the fight and may even encourage your husband to talk about *his* contributions.

If you know all these things, you can't possibly relate to your husband in the same old way; you will *automatically* be having a different relationship with him. *That's* how knowing these principles is using them.

Skeptic: Well, I think I get the idea. But why can't I go further and use them *concretely*—you know, by deciding to make "I statements" rather than "you statements," by deciding to talk about only my contribution to the fight, by just—

Wile: Because you can't just *decide* to make "I statements" rather than "you statements"; they won't come out right. They'll sound awkward or not quite believable—or they'll be "you statements" in disguise. To make "I statements" that are really "I statements" and have the best chance of being heard as such, you've got to be in the right state of mind. The same holds true for just *deciding* to talk about only your contribution to the fight. You've got to be in the right state of mind for that too. And the only way to be in the right state of mind is for your husband to talk about only *his* contribution to the fight, so *he's* got to be in the right state of mind at the same time.

CHAPTER 19

The "Collaborating–Collaborating" Couple State

Marie is amazed that Paul has actually come to her and tried to talk about the fight. She cannot remember the last time he did something like that—she thinks it was never. And Paul's efforts are actually working out. She and Paul are in the "admitting–admitting" couple state. But how have they gotten there? By means of a long and complex process. Marie and Paul have passed through a number of couple states this evening:

- *The "overwhelmed–abandoned" couple state.* Paul, feeling overwhelmed by Marie's immediately meeting him after work with a complete report of her bad day, escaped to watch the News, leaving Marie in the hallway feeling abandoned.

- *The "seeking-privacy–feeling-rejected" couple state.* While Paul was in front of the TV seeking a moment of privacy, Marie was making dinner feeling rejected.

- *The "adversarial–adversarial" couple state.* Marie stormed into the living room and said, "You never talk to me any more." Paul defended himself, and the fight was on.

- *The "hit-and-run-perpetrator–hit-and-run-victim" couple state.* Paul called Marie a nag and disappeared into the rain.

- *The "peace-offering–peace-rejecting" couple state.* Marie, still smarting from the hit-and-run, rejected Paul's initial peace overture.

- *The return of the "adversarial–adversarial" couple state.* Frustrated by the rejection of his peace-offer, Paul snapped at Marie, rekindling the fight.

- *The "licking-wounds–licking-wounds" couple state.* Paul escaped to lick his wounds, leaving Marie to do the same.

193

• *The "admitting–admitting" couple state.* In a renewed peace-making attempt, Paul admitted that his calling Marie a nag was a low blow. His admission led ultimately to a new couple state in which each partner's willingness to admit his or her contribution to the problem led the other to feel like making a similar admission.

So Marie and Paul are presently in the "admitting–admitting" couple state. This state is delicately balanced, and there is little room for error. Any comment by either partner that strikes the other as containing even a touch of blame can upset the balance, snapping them back into an "adversarial–adversarial" state. The only way for them to talk about their fight without rekindling it is for each to talk about his or her own—but not the other's—contribution to it.

There is, however, another couple state—the "collaborating–collaborating" couple state—that is *not* so delicately balanced and in which there *is* room for error. It is a couple state in which it *is* possible to talk about the other's contribution to the fight without immediately rekindling it. And it is into this state that Paul and Marie are about to shift.

Paul's "I had a bad day at work, and I guess I took it out on you" made Marie feel he was willing to look at things from her point of view. Marie's "I know I can come on pretty strong" made Paul feel that she was willing to look at things from *his* point of view. The cumulative effect of such admissions is a buildup of good will. By slow degrees, the "admitting–admitting" couple state has led them to the "collaborating–collaborating" couple state.

Earlier, when Marie was in the "adversarial" state, she looked for hidden barbs in even seemingly friendly comments. Now, in the "collaborating" state, she doesn't expect a barb. And if she finds one, she is likely to attribute it to a momentary irritation of Paul's rather than to deep-seated resentment, which is how she would see it if she were still in the "adversarial" state. Now if Paul says something that hits her a bit wrong, Marie automatically assumes that it wasn't meant to hurt, in contrast to the "adversarial" state, in which she would automatically assume his hateful feelings and bad intentions.

The shift to the "collaborating–collaborating" state means that it is now possible for Marie or Paul to refer to the other's contribution to the fight, and even be a little accusing, without immediately rekindling the fight. Because of the good will accumulated while in the "admitting–admitting" state, there is some margin for error.

Which is a good thing, because what Paul says next *does* seem to Marie a little accusing:

I've been under attack from every direction these days.

Marie wonders whether Paul includes *her* among the attackers.

If Marie and Paul were in the "adversarial–adversarial" couple state, she would say, "You always think I'm attacking you when I'm not, and you have the nerve to call *me* oversensitive."

If Marie and Paul were in the "admitting–admitting" couple state, she would say, "I feel bad because I don't support you as much as I should; in fact, sometimes I *am* one of the attackers."

But Marie and Paul are in the "collaborating–collaborating" couple state, so she says:

> I'm worried that you count *me* as one of the attackers. Do you?

If Marie and Paul were in the "adversarial–adversarial" couple state, Paul would say, "You always think I'm criticizing you when I'm not; you *are* oversensitive."

If Marie and Paul were in the "admitting–admitting" couple state, he would say, "I know I shouldn't see you as attacking; you're only trying to help."

Since they are in the "collaborating–collaborating" couple state, Paul says:

> Well, I *do* sometimes count you as one of the attackers. But other times—like now—I feel you're on my side.

If they were in the "adversarial–adversarial" couple state, Marie would say, "We're never going to get anywhere as long as you insist that I'm attacking you."

In the "admitting–admitting" couple state . . . well, Marie and Paul would probably no longer be in that state. As I said, being in the "admitting–admitting" state means having little margin for error. What Paul just said could easily have pushed Marie over the line.

But Marie and Paul are in the "collaborating–collaborating" couple state. So she says:

> Well, I guess sometimes I *am* one of the attackers. I can't stand the idea that I'm getting to be like my mother, who was always attacking my father. Come to think of it, you remind me a little of him when you react by immediately escaping.

Being in the "collaborating–collaborating" couple state means that Marie is not just accusing Paul of things (the "adversarial–adversarial" couple state) and Marie is not just admitting things (the "admitting–

admitting" couple state). She is standing back, looking at both herself and Paul, and reporting her feelings and reactions whatever they are. Snapping into the "collaborating–collaborating" state is, in this sense, getting on the joint platform.

Paul is not happy with what Marie is reporting, however:

> I'm not at all like your father.

Comparing Paul to her father is not crucial to Marie's point. What is crucial is that she is worried that she is like her mother. Saying that Paul is like her father was just an afterthought.

But Paul's defensive response, which indicates that he has just snapped into the "adversarial" state, snaps Marie into it too. And being in the "adversarial" state, Marie forgets that telling Paul he is like her father was not crucial to her point.

But it is crucial now. What had been an afterthought a moment ago, when Marie was in the "collaborating" state, has become the central point now. And now we see why partners get stuck arguing about irrelevant matters, such as whether a specific event occurred *before* Thanksgiving or *after* Thanksgiving. Once partners shift to the "adversarial–adversarial" state, *everything* becomes a bone of contention.

Since Marie and Paul are momentarily in the "adversarial–adversarial" couple state, Marie answers Paul's "I'm not at all like your father" with this:

> You're *exactly* like him. Precisely at six every night, he'd disappear to watch the News, leaving my mom to take care of everything. How is that different from what you did tonight?

Has the collaborating spirit disappeared?

Not *entirely*. The good will that was built up a little while ago exerts a moderating force. Without this good will, Paul would probably have said at this point, "Well, you'd hardly blame him. He'd need a storm cellar to protect himself against your mother; I could use one myself." And that would really get Marie going. As a result of the buildup of good will, however, Paul does not counterattack so harshly. Instead, he simply defends himself, which is a less provocative response. He points out how he is *not* like Marie's father:

> You said it yourself—your father did it every night. I just do it once in a while. And he'd stay plastered to the tube till it was time for bed, and I just watch the News.

The cache of good will exerts a moderating force on Marie, too. Without it, she would probably have said, "So? Do you want a gold star?" Which would be hard for *Paul* to take. But because of the buildup of good will, she says:

> Well, I *still* don't like it. But you're right. That *is* a difference—and I have to admit, it's a big one.

Marie has moved back in the direction of a collaborating state, and Paul follows her:

> Well, I appreciate your saying it.

The "collaborating–collaborating" couple state that Marie and Paul experienced a few minutes ago thus provides a cushion of good will that protects them from snapping too firmly back into the "adversarial–adversarial" state. And if they *do* momentarily return to it (as they just did), they can more easily snap out of it.

CHAPTER 20

A Recovery Conversation in Its Full Sense

E veryone's first choice, of course, is not to have fights at all. Unfortunately, people do not always get their first choice. Periods of irritability, misunderstanding, and not seeing eye to eye are inevitable; that is, there are always going to be fights. If these fights are not out in the open, they are going to be under the table—with cutting looks, angry silences, and sarcastic remarks.

Since there are always going to be fights, I recommend developing skill in recovering from them. One way of recovering is having conversations like those described in the last several chapters.

Recovery conversations are chancy. They can rekindle the fight. But they have several important advantages over all the other methods of recovery (methods such as "apologizing and saying no more about it" or "going on as if nothing has happened"). They can:

1. Lead to a sense of resolution about the fight.
2. Produce a sense of intimacy.
3. Plumb the fight for whatever information it may reveal about the relationship.

The purpose of this chapter is to discuss these three special advantages of recovery conversations.

A Sense of Resolution about the Fight

Marie and Paul's attempt to talk about their fight tonight has gone fairly well. They shifted first from an "adversarial–adversarial" to an "admitting–admitting" and then to a "collaborating–collaborating" couple state.

And after snapping back briefly into "adversarial–adversarial," they have now returned to a "collaborating–collaborating" state. Marie has just admitted that Paul is not entirely like her father—her father would stay glued to the TV all evening, whereas Paul just watches the News. Paul appreciates Marie's recognizing this difference. And Marie appreciates his appreciation.

To demonstrate that she harbors no ill will—and in an effort to eliminate any residual ill will on Paul's part—Marie now says:

> Of course, on nights like this, when everything goes wrong, maybe we'd do better to follow in Dad's tradition: Maybe both of us should stare at the tube all evening without saying a word.

Marie's hope is that Paul will take her joke in the positive spirit she means it.

PAUL: Not a bad idea—tonight was certainly not the best time we ever spent together.
MARIE: On a scale from 1 to 10, I'd give it a 3.
PAUL: Too high. I'd say 1½ is more like it.

Paul's willingness to go along with her attempt to lighten the mood convinces Marie that he harbors no ill will. He has joined her in the "playful–playful, willing-to-joke-about-it" couple state.

MARIE: *That* bad, huh?
PAUL: That bad, yes.
MARIE: Of course, we had two strikes against us. Each of us came home black and blue from work. I had a horrible day, and, if I get you right, you did too.

In saying that they each had horrible days, Marie is beginning to talk about the fight—or, at least, about what led up to it. And that is a bit chancy, since talking about the fight can easily rekindle it. Paul's joining her in the "playful–playful, willing-to-joke-about-it" couple state has emboldened her, however.

And Marie's "I had a horrible day, and, if I get you right, you did too" does *not* rekindle the fight. Instead of blaming Paul, which *would* start it up again, Marie is sympathizing with him for having had a bad day. And at the same time, Marie is sympathizing with herself for having had a bad day too.

And the fact that Marie is not blaming Paul emboldens *him* to talk about the fight:

And we did what we usually do when we come home from work in a foul mood: You wanted to talk and I wanted time to myself—so we found ourselves completely at odds. Strike three.

Paul is suggesting, in essence, that it is a shame that Marie wanted to talk when he wanted time to himself—and it is a shame that he wanted time to himself when Marie wanted to talk. Marie replies:

Marie: And I complained that you never talk to me and you called me a nag. Strike four.

Marie has now said the "N" word—"nag." And that sets off an alarm in Paul. He is worried that Marie may still be angry at him for that. So he changes the subject:

You don't know much about baseball, do you? There is no "strike four."

But Marie changes it back:

There is the way *we* play it. We keep missing the ball—and each other. You tried to reach out after the fight, but I wasn't ready.

Since Marie clearly is not angry at him, Paul rejoins the effort to talk about the fight:

PAUL: And that got me frustrated. I called you a bump on a log.
MARIE: Then *I* got frustrated. I said, "Well, I didn't ask you to come in here." At least I *think* that's what I said. When I get really mad, it's hard to remember what I say.
PAUL: That's how I remember it too. Then we went off and spent the next hour nursing our wounds.

So Marie and Paul are talking about the fight, and in a "not-blaming, sympathizing-with-each-other" way. That is, they are on the joint platform, sympathizing:

With *Paul* for having had a horrible day, for not getting time for himself, for being criticized for not talking, and for having his peace overture rejected.
With *Marie* for having had a horrible day, for not getting a chance to talk, for being called a nag, and for having to deal with Paul's frustration when she refused to accept his peace overture.

This is how Marie and Paul achieve a sense of resolution about the fight: by arriving together at a "nonblaming, we-just-got-stuck-in-something" sense of how they got into the fight—or rather, by moving into a couple state that allows them to arrive at this picture. To do so, they have had to pass through:

The "admitting–admitting" couple state.

The "collaborating–collaborating" couple state.

The "playful–playful, willing-to-joke-about-it" couple state.

The "what-a-shame-it-had-to-happen–what-a-shame-it-had-to-happen" couple state, which is a special form of the "collaborating–collaborating" couple state.

The good will generated by each of these states has moved them into the next. At any moment, however, the tide could have turned. A comment by either could have been experienced by the other as an attack and started things moving back in the "adversarial–adversarial" direction.

But the tide has *not* turned. In fact, the good will generated by the "what-a-shame-it-had-to-happen–what-a-shame-it-had-to-happen" couple state is about to snap Marie and Paul into an even more desirable couple state: the "feeling-touched–feeling-touched" couple state.

A Sense of Intimacy: The "Feeling-Touched–Feeling-Touched" Couple State

Marie and Paul have just described how, following Paul's "Don't just sit there like a bump on a log" and Marie's "I didn't ask you to come in here," both went off to lick their wounds. Marie comments:

I was surprised we came out of it at all. I thought we'd do what we usually do after a fight: spend the rest of the evening ignoring each other, and climb into bed as if the other person weren't in it.

In saying, ". . . climb into bed as if the other person weren't in it," Marie is putting something new into words. She is extending the area of shared awareness. She is claiming for her and Paul as a couple this experience that each has previously been struggling with alone. She is taking Paul into her confidence, making this experience something about which they can jointly commiserate. She is making him an ally in her struggle with him.

And Paul responds by taking Marie into *his* confidence and by making *her* an ally:

PAUL: Yes, I never get much sleep on those nights.

MARIE: Me neither. And sometimes in the middle of the night, I wake up feeling lonely and want to cuddle. But I don't want to be the first to give in, so I just lie there hoping you'll reach over. And you never do.

PAUL: No—because *I* don't want to be the one to give in. So I just lie there hoping you'll make the first move.

MARIE: Pretty ridiculous, isn't it?

Marie and Paul are in the "confiding–confiding, feeling-safe-with-each-other" couple state, which enables Paul to become aware of something that he can only notice when he *is* feeling particularly safe with Marie:

> You know, I really took it hard when you complained that I never talk to you any more. It shocked me.

In place of the "hard-shell, self-protective, refusing-to-admit-that-anything-Marie-said-got-to-me" attitude with which Paul originally greeted Marie's "You never talk to me any more," Paul is now exposing his soft underbelly: "I took your criticism hard; it shocked me." Marie is immediately disarmed. Instead of moving in for the kill, she throws down her weapons:

MARIE: It shocked *me*. I didn't know I was going to say it. It just slipped out.

PAUL: But did you mean it? I'd hate it if you thought of me as one of those grim, silent husbands who relates to the TV better than to his wife.

Marie hesitates—she fears that Paul is not going to like what she is about to say. But she says it anyway. Now, she thinks, is not the time to be evasive:

> Well, I guess I do sometimes—at least I did tonight. A lot of upsetting things happened today, and I really needed to talk.

Paul feels bad that he did not talk. He snaps into the "self-accusing" state—which he deals with by immediately snapping into the "accusing-Marie, it's-her-own-fault-for-not-telling-me" defensive state:

> If that's what you wanted, why didn't you tell me?

Paul is defending himself with Response 19: **You should have told me.**

MARIE: I *couldn't* tell you. I'd only just figured it out myself.
PAUL: Well, how could you expect *me* to figure it out then? I'm not a magician.

If it were not for the good will that has built up between them, Marie would be likely to say something like "It wouldn't take a magician to figure out I needed a little understanding." Because of the good will, however, she is able to listen to Paul's charge without completely losing her sense of humor:

Well, a little magic wouldn't hurt at a time like this.

That Marie does not take offense at what Paul has just said is all he needs to regain *his* sense of humor:

I used up all my magic at the store. You can't imagine what *I* had to deal with today.

Paul's regaining his sense of humor is all Marie needs to recover her "feeling-safe-with-Paul" state of mind—which, in turn, is all she needs to become aware of what she really wanted from him tonight:

MARIE: Well, that's too bad, because after magically figuring out that I needed some understanding and cheering up, you were supposed to magically figure out what else was on my mind.
PAUL: There was *more*?
MARIE: Isn't there always? I wanted us to spend the evening planning wonderful vacations that would take me away from all of this.

If this is what Marie wanted with Paul tonight, why didn't she tell him earlier? Because in order to tell him what she wanted—or even just to know what it is—she has to be in the "feeling-safe-with-Paul, feeling-cared-for-and-sympathized-with-by-him" state of mind. Paul's warm comments, which are in themselves comforting and revitalizing, snap her into such state of mind; that is, they enable her to recognize the full extent of the comforting and revitalizing she wants.

Marie is telling Paul what she really wanted from him tonight—and without criticizing him for not providing it. By saying that he was "magically" supposed to figure out what she wanted, she is admitting that it was unrealistic of her to expect that he could. She is letting Paul off the hook.

And, let off the hook, Paul can listen to what Marie says—and sympathize with her about it. Instead of criticizing her for expecting him to magically solve her problems, Paul makes an equivalent admission:

PAUL: Well, it's funny you're saying that, because it reminds me of something I'd completely forgotten until right now. I hoped you would somehow know that I had a horrible day and say something to make me feel better.
MARIE: I don't believe it—not *you*!

It's too *good* to believe. Marie cannot imagine that Paul—the original "I've-got-it-all-covered, superguy, I-can-handle-it-all-myself" person—would actually need her to help him out of a funk.

Paul, even more than Marie, feels uncomfortable with needing something from another to help him feel better. He *too* feels unentitled to these wishes—which is why he had forgotten them.

MARIE: Now, tell the truth. What you *really* wanted was to be left alone.
PAUL: Well, sure, when I first got home. But later I would have liked some company. In fact, talking about vacations would have been fun.
MARIE: I still can't believe what you're saying.
PAUL: I can't either—it doesn't sound like me. But it *is* what I was feeling.

Marie's eyes well up with tears; it really *is* too good to believe. She often feels that Paul doesn't want anything from her—that he just sees her as a necessary cog in the running of the house, or, worse, simply as a pest. So she is touched by the realization that he *does* want something from her—and that it's the same thing that she wants from him. That is why Marie is on the verge of crying: She feels less alone. And, feeling less alone, she becomes aware of how alone she *has* been feeling—and now she really wants to cry.

At its best, a recovery conversation can:

- Make you feel understood.
- Produce a sense of safety and good will.
- Make you feel less alone.
- Repair the damage caused by the fight.
- Produce a sense of connectedness and rapprochement.
- Make you aware of just how alone, misunderstood, unsafe, and unconnected you have been feeling.

In brief, it can snap you into the "feeling-intimate–feeling-intimate" couple state of mind.

Plumbing the Fight for Useful Information about the Relationship

I have discussed the first two of the three special advantages that recovery conversations have over other methods of recovery: (1) establishing a sense of resolution about the fight, and (2) providing a greater sense of intimacy. I now turn to the third: (3) plumbing the fight for whatever useful information it may reveal about the relationship.

We all know that people often say things in fights that they don't mean. We also know that only in fights, when all the constraints are off, are people sometimes finally freed to say what they *do* mean. Unfortunately, the attacking, exaggerated, distorted, blurted-out manner in which each person says these things makes it difficult for the other to hear them.

That is where the recovery conversation comes in. After the fight, when partners are no longer in the "adversarial–adversarial" couple state, it is possible to go back over what was said and tap the fight for whatever information it might reveal about the relationship.

PAUL: Did you really mean it when you said, "You never talk to me any more?"
MARIE: Well, I did *sort* of mean it. I was frustrated, so I exaggerated a little. I was upset that you didn't talk to me tonight. I wanted us to be close; I wanted us to spend some time cuddled up on the couch, talking vacation talk.

Marie and Paul's recovery conversation has thus revealed that her "You never talk to me any more" was an angry, exaggerated, blurted-out way of saying that she was disappointed that Paul didn't listen to her, cheer her up, and fantasize about their running off together.

Now that she is able to state this wish, it enables Paul to discover that he often has a similar one:

You know, I think there are *lots* of times that I come home thinking I don't want anything from you when actually I do.

This is an example of how Marie and Paul can use a recovery conversation to plumb the fight for useful information about the relationship. Paul has discovered a wish that neither he nor Marie previously knew he had. Marie has discovered that he doesn't really want to shut her out when he comes home, even if he acts as if he does.

Skeptic: But look how hard it was, all the cleverness and luck it took to make it work out. I'd hate to have to count on that all the time.

Wile: Yes, and that's why most couples don't even try to have recovery conversations.

Skeptic: And I don't blame them. I know I'm contradicting myself— again—but again I'm thinking that it's too risky to talk about a fight. It's too easy for something to go wrong. It's too seldom that a couple has the kind of recovery conversation you've just described.

Wile: Well, you're right, of course, although it's a shame you are, because without such recovery conversations:

> There is no chance to discover what the fight was really about.
> There is no chance to discover what the fight is revealing about the relationship.
> There will be a buildup of unresolved interactions taking their toll on the relationship—with each unresolved fight adding an additional increment of alienation.

Accordingly, when I see people in couples therapy, I try to give them a taste of a recovery conversation.

Implications for Therapy

So that is how it might look if Marie and Paul were to have a full-fledged recovery conversation. Of course, as the author of this book, I have *arranged* for them to have it. I want to describe the difficulties partners encounter in their attempts at such conversations, and to demonstrate certain principles that explain these difficulties. Ordinarily Marie and Paul would not even attempt such a conversation. They would just be relieved that the fight was over. They wouldn't want to talk about the fight and risk rekindling it.

One of the things I try to do in therapy is to give couples experiences with recovery conversations that work out—or at least work out better than the ones they might have on their own. And I do this by making framing statements and by stating left-out feelings.

Framing Statements

Here are examples of framing and prefacing statements that partners typically exclude from their conversations—and whose exclusion can easily transform their conversations into fights:

Instead of saying, "Our conversation has just taken a sour turn and I'm worried that we're about to get back into the fight," partners just blurt out, "There you go again . . ."

Instead of saying, "I'm afraid you might take this as an attack—and, come to think of it, maybe it is; I am kind of angry—but mostly I just want to get some things off my chest. And it's that . . . ," they just go ahead and attack. They say, "You never . . ."

Instead of saying, "I'm worried that you might think this is unfair—in fact, it probably is—but I feel that . . . ," they say, "Do you always have to . . . ?"

Instead of saying, "I know this isn't going to come out right—I've been sitting on it and I've built up a lot of steam—but . . . ," they go full steam ahead and open the vent. They say, "Why do you always have to . . . ?"

Instead of saying, "I know I'm being defensive, but . . . ," they just act defensive. They say, "You're wrong. And anyway, you do the same thing yourself. And furthermore . . ."

Instead of saying, "I did those things for you just because I wanted to—with no strings attached, expecting nothing in return—but, for some reason, now I find myself suddenly *resenting* you for not doing anything in return," they say, "It would never occur to you to do something nice for me once in a while."

Instead of saying, "I know that by repeating the point in this angry way I'm only making things worse—it's not going to get you to listen—but I'm feeling too frustrated to stop," they just go ahead and repeat the point.

Left-Out Feelings

The first six of the seven principles for helping partners have recovery conversations are based on left-out feelings. Their purpose, in fact, is to draw attention to feelings that, as a result of being left out, rekindle the fight:

The point of Principle 1 (the "'I-statements'-versus-'you-statements'" principle) is that, if you leave out feelings ("I statements") and instead make accusations ("you statements"), you are likely to rekindle the fight.

The point of Principle 2 (the "taking-your-partner's-point-of-view" principle) is that your partner needs you to appreciate his or her feelings before being able to appreciate yours.

The point of Principle 3 (the "nice-guy-backlash" principle) is that problems arise when you are unable to confide in your partner that you are feeling taken advantage of or taken for granted. You

resent going the extra mile and feeling that the other is not reciprocating or even sufficiently appreciating.

The point of Principle 4 (the "expecting-to-rekindle-the-fight" principle) is that problems arise when you are unable to confide in
your partner about your rekindled angry feelings and, instead, just
say angry things.

The point of Principle 5 (the "looking-for-the-missing-piece" principle) is that the reason your partner is not coming around is that
something is stuck in his or her craw; that is, there are feelings
that he or she needs to figure out and express.

The point of Principle 6 (the "two-conflicting-missing-pieces" principle) is that something is stuck in both your craws—which is what
maintains the fight. In other words, there are feelings that *each*
partner needs to figure out and express.

Inserting These Omitted Elements in Therapy

As I have said earlier, I try to give partners an experience of a more successful recovery conversation than the ones they are able to have on
their own. I do so largely by inserting both left-out feelings and excluded
framing statements. Let us suppose that Marie and Paul are in my office
when they have the conversation described in this section of the book.
Marie has just said:

> I can't stand the idea that you're getting to be like my father, who
> continually withdrew.

> To which Paul replies:

PAUL: I'm not at all like your father.
THERAPIST (*to Paul*): I imagine that, hearing what Marie just said, you
might feel hurt.

> I have inserted what I guess is Paul's feeling.

PAUL: Well, I wouldn't say "hurt"—that puts it a little strong . . . well,
actually, maybe I *do* feel hurt. I'd hate to think that Marie really
sees me as her father. I know how he always let her down.
MARIE (*turning to Paul*): Well, you act like him sometimes. Do you want
me to pretend that you don't?

> Marie is defending herself by insisting that she is simply reporting
the truth. My guess, knowing Marie, is that she is defending herself

because she feels bad about hurting Paul. The important feeling she is leaving out is that she feels bad. My task is to insert this left-out feeling. I try to think of a way to do so that she will accept, even *enjoy*.

THERAPIST (*to Marie*): I wonder if you feel—here, I'll be you talking to Paul, and I'll say, "Paul, I feel bad that you feel hurt—I don't want to hurt you. I just want you to see that sometimes I can feel with you what I used to feel all the time with my dad."
MARIE (*relieved*): *Yes*, that says it.

I may continue back and forth between Marie and Paul several times, inserting left-out feelings and excluded framing statements. Why do I do that? Why do I place such emphasis on these omitted elements? I insert them:

> To give Marie and Paul the chance to have a *conversation*. Without the tempering effect of these inserted elements, the fight would quickly drown out the conversation.
> To show Marie and Paul how to have a conversation about touchy matters. I don't expect them to go home and be able to have such conversations on their own immediately, but I hope a little of it will rub off.
> To introduce Marie and Paul to the idea of left-out feelings and excluded framing statements (in fact, this is my major purpose). I want to give them the advantage of knowing that their problems in talking (and thinking) are the result of leaving out these feelings and statements.

I want to give Marie and Paul a working familiarity with the "problems-are-the-result-of-left-out-feelings-and-omitted-framing-statements" principle by demonstrating it in action. I want them to develop a familiarity with the couple states they are likely to go through when they try to talk about their fights. I want them to have a bird's-eye view of the states they go in and out of—ideally, *as* they go in and out of them. I want them to have a supraordinate couple state—yes, a platform—from which they can jointly observe all these other states. I want them to be conversant with these states and conversant with one another about them.

> I want them to know about the "adversarial–adversarial" couple state: to be able to recognize when they are in it, and to appreciate that any attempt to talk about the fight at such times will become part of the fight.
> I want them to know about the "admitting–admitting" couple state: how it persists only as long as each talks solely about his or her contribution to the fight.

I want them to know about the "collaborating–collaborating" couple state, in which the buildup of good will allows them a certain margin for error in talking about the fight.

I want them to know about "I statements versus you statements," "nice-guy backlash," "something stuck in their craws," and all the other principles.

One way I inform couples about their couple states is to make up conversations for them that reveal these states:

If they are presently in the "adversarial–adversarial" couple state, I may show them the conversation they might have if they were in the "admitting–admitting" couple state—in the process, making clear to them the nature of both couple states.

If they are presently in the "admitting–admitting" couple state, I may show them the conversation they might have if they were in the "adversarial–adversarial" couple state—again demonstrating the character of both states.

My goal—often unachievable—is to enable partners to have the particular interaction they are having—that is, to fully inhabit their present couple state—and, at the same time (or some time afterward), to imagine the conversation they could be having were they in another state.

In describing Marie and Paul's evening, I have emphasized "states of mind." In this chapter, I have introduced the idea of "left-out feelings" and the related notion of "omitted framing statements." In the following chapters, I show how Marie and Paul's whole evening can be looked at as the consequence of left-out feelings and omitted framing statements.

PART 6

THE NEED TO GET SOMETHING ACROSS

We have discovered in the previous chapter that Paul had a day-dream that Marie would cheer him up after his difficult day, but he wasn't able to tell her about it because he thought he shouldn't have it. This discovery opens up a new way of looking at Marie and Paul's evening—and at couple life in general:

Marie and Paul's (and every couple's) problems result from an inability to talk to each other about certain feelings because they feel unentitled to them (Chapters 21 and 22).

Relationships provide a built-in person to help each partner deal with feelings to which he or she feels unentitled. But rather than helping, this built-in person may echo the taskmaster's charges and increase the partner's feeling of unentitlement (Chapter 23).

Therapy is devoted to figuring out the crucial feeling to which, at any given moment, each client feels unentitled, and recognizing the extent to which partners function as confidants to each other in dealing with these feelings (Chapter 24).

Communication skills training can be thought of, in part, as an effort to help partners fulfill their potential to be confidants in dealing with feelings to which they feel unentitled (Chapter 25).

CHAPTER 21

Leading-Edge Feelings

It turns out that Paul had the same wish Marie had—he, too, wanted to be cheered up after a difficult day. That is what their recovery conversation has revealed. But how can knowing this help?

It can help because *not* knowing this is what led to the problem in the first place. When we are unable to get across our leading-edge, major-and-immediate, top-of-the-mind feelings, we generate symptoms. That is the point of this chapter: to show how not knowing about your feelings and wishes—and not being able to get them across to your partner—is a major source of couple problems.

Let us go back in time and imagine a different set of circumstances. Let us imagine what would happen if Paul were to feel sufficiently entitled to his wish that Marie comfort him that, when she greets him at the door, he is able to say:

> You know, on the way home, I had this incredible fantasy that you'd know the kind of day I'd had. As soon as I came in the door, you'd start taking care of me, do all sorts of comforting, distracting, wonderful things. I feel foolish telling you about it, though. How could you guess that I had a horrible day? And besides, maybe your day wasn't much better, and you might need *me* to comfort *you.*

If Paul were able to say that, Marie might be able to say:

> Well, I *did* have a horrible day—so I guess we'll need to comfort one another.

And the whole evening would go differently:

- Paul would bring into the open that he wants comforting; he would be confiding in Marie rather than withdrawing from her.
- And Marie, seeing that Paul wants something from her—and that he is confiding in her—would not feel so alone.
- And since Paul's comment would draw from Marie that she, too, wants comforting, he would be helping her confide in him.
- And Paul would not have to listen to Marie's laundry list of her bad day without hearing the main point, which is that she wants comforting. She would supply this point; his telling her that he wants comforting would draw from her that *she* does too.
- And the comforting would already be beginning—since Paul and Marie would be confiding in each other. To a large extent, that is what comforting is.

And now we can appreciate Paul's disadvantage in not being able to tell Marie about his daydream. Instead of comforting and being comforted, confiding and being confided in, Paul stands there alienated from Marie—and, more importantly, from himself. He is cut off from his wish to be comforted—it has never fully registered—because he feels he shouldn't have it. He feels *unentitled* to it. He thinks it is babyish to expect Marie to drop everything and attend to his needs. He is in the "not-approving-of-what's-on-my-mind-and-so-not-knowing-what-it-is, cut-off-from-myself, not-having-anything-to-say" alienated state.

Since Paul has nothing to say, Marie steps into the breach. She *does* have something to say. She tells Paul how the kids misbehaved and about her problems at work. But she is not much better able to tell Paul about her wish to be comforted than Paul is able to tell her about his. She doesn't feel any more entitled to these wishes than Paul does. The closest she can come is to detail the problems of her day, secretly hoping that his response will be to comfort her. Without hearing the main point—that is, without hearing why she is telling him this, that, and the other—Paul feels flooded by the details.

A minute ago, coming up the walk, Paul was in a "Marie-is-a-resource, she-can-comfort-me" state of mind. As a result of this brief interchange, he now snaps into a "Marie-is-a-burden, I've-got-to-get-out-of-here" state. All Paul can think of at the moment is how to get away. What is amazing is what Paul does *not* say to himself:

> What's happening? This is incredible. A minute ago I was looking forward to seeing Marie. Now she's become a major problem I have to *cope* with. How can that be? How can things change so fast?

Why *doesn't* Paul say this to himself? He is so used to such shifts—they are so much a part of his everyday life—that he hardly notices them. All he knows is that he wants to put some distance between himself and the "major problem."

So he makes an excuse and disappears to watch the News.

Intimacy Is Always Just a Sentence Away

Sitting in front of the TV set, Paul feels bad about letting Marie down. She clearly wants to talk. He worries that something is wrong with him for not wanting to listen. He worries that maybe he is too detached, that he is incapable of having an intimate relationship.

He does not know it, but he has just passed through a series of four alienated states:

- The "losing-track-of-my-daydream, not-knowing-what's-on-my-mind, not-having-anything-to-say" alienated state.
- The "feeling-flooded, why-does-Marie-have-to-carry-on-this-way" alienated state.
- The "I-can't-stand-this, I've-got-to-get-out-of-here" alienated state.
- The "blaming-myself, feeling-bad-about-letting-Marie-down" alienated state.

Being in an alienated state means being disconnected from your leading-edge feeling. At any given moment, there is always such a feeling. To begin at the beginning of this sequence, Paul's leading-edge feeling as he walks in the door is his wish that Marie know he'd had a horrible day and be wonderfully comforting.

But Paul is unable to put this feeling into words—even to himself. He feels unentitled to it. So he just stands there, at a loss, not knowing what he feels, not knowing what to say—with Marie looking at him expectantly. And that means that he now has a new leading-edge feeling that he needs (but is unable) to express to Marie:

I feel at a loss. I know there was something that I wanted to tell you, but I can't seem to pin it down. My mind is a total blank.

The fact that Paul is alienated from his leading-edge feeling of wanting Marie to comfort him means that he is immediately confronted by a *new* leading-edge feeling: the feeling of alienation from his original feeling.

If Paul were able to express this new feeling—if he could tell Marie that he feels alienated and at a loss—he would be bringing her in on his alienated state. He would be shifting from the "not-knowing-what's-on-my-mind" alienated state to the *"confiding-in-Marie-about-not-knowing-what's-on-my-mind" intimate* state. He would be connecting with Marie about how he is disconnected from himself. By getting Marie to notice that there is something he wants to tell her (even if he cannot remember what it is), he would be getting a taste of what he wanted in the first place: Marie's attention to his feelings.

Of course, he is even less likely to be able to tell Marie about his "my-mind-is-a-total-blank" feeling than to tell her about his "as-I-came-up-the-walk-I-had-this-incredible-fantasy" feeling. That is because it does not seem like a feeling at all. And when Marie, stepping into the breach, tells him about the problems of *her* day, there is immediately a new leading-edge feeling he needs to express to Marie in order to stop feeling alienated from her. He needs to tell her:

> I hate what I'm feeling—and I hate myself for feeling it—but all I can think of right now is that I want to get away. And I'm worried about what it means that I'm not even willing to listen to you when you've had a bad day. I feel like a total failure as a husband.

In saying this, Paul would be bringing Marie in on his alienated state. He would be shifting from the "feeling-like-a-total-failure-for-wanting-to-get-away" alienated state to the *"confiding*-in-Marie-about-my-feeling-like-a-total-failure-for-wanting-to-get-away" intimate state.

But Paul is too worried about being a total failure to be able to stand back and talk about it. Instead of telling Marie that he needs to get away—and that he feels bad about this need—he just *gets* away. He makes an excuse and escapes to the living room. That immediately puts him in a position where there is a new leading-edge feeling he needs to get across to Marie in order to stop feeling alienated from her. He needs to tell her:

> I thought that going in to watch the News would help. But it isn't. I'm just sitting here, staring at the tube, feeling lousy about skipping out when I knew you wanted to talk.

In saying this, Paul would be bringing Marie in on his alienated state. He would be shifting from the "feeling-down, self-critical" alienated state to the *"confiding-in-Marie-*about-feeling-down, self-critical" *intimate* state.

But Paul is unable to say this, just as he has been unable to make any of the previous statements. Instead, he just sinks deeper and deeper into an alienated state. But no matter how deep he gets, he can *still* at any moment break out of it, simply by confiding in Marie about the state he is in.

My point here is that intimacy is always just a sentence away—even though you might not be able to think of the sentence. And alienation is always just the *lack* of this sentence away. And now it is clear what lies at the root of Marie and Paul's (and everyone's) problems: alienation caused by the inability to come up with the necessary sentence.

Since much of the time it will be impossible to get across what you need to, you are going to be alienated much of the time. Being human means being alienated much of the time, although we are all so used to it—alienation is so much a part of everyday life—that we typically ignore it. We do not usually think of ourselves as alienated.

At any moment Paul can shift out of his alienated state, simply by letting Marie in on it. But letting Marie in on it is not something he would ordinarily think to do.

So Marie and Paul's evenings—and everyone's—are typically a succession of alienated states with, on the better evenings, a few intimate states thrown in. In the version of events presented earlier in this book, tonight was actually one of those better evenings. Marie's marching into the living room and telling Paul, "You never talk to me any more," which provoked a fight, led to an intimate interaction later on.

Generating Symptoms

Let us imagine how this evening might have gone if Marie had not said what she had; the fight had not taken place; and, as a result, they had not had that intimate interaction. Let us imagine that on the way to the living room, Marie smells something burning and rushed back to the kitchen. She never makes it to the living room. Instead of storming at Paul for not talking to her, she storms at herself for burning the rice:

Damn—it's completely ruined!

And that means that there is a new leading-edge feeling that *Marie* needs to be able to get across in order to avoid feeling alienated from Paul. She needs to be able to say to him:

The rice is the last straw. I'm standing here in front of a pot full of inedible muck, feeling miserable and alone, wanting to reach out to you, but not knowing how to do it without making things worse.

Marie's "Damn—it's completely ruined!", which she says loud enough for Paul to hear in the living room, is a symptomatic act. It is the result of her inability to get across what she needs to and her frustrated substitute effort to express it. She hopes Paul will come into the kitchen and show his concern.

But Paul does *not* come in. Instead, he sits tight and generates symptoms of his own. In fact, staying where he is, not paying attention to Marie's outcry, and continuing to watch TV are themselves symptoms.

I know that when we use the word "symptoms" we typically think of maladaptive or pathological reactions such as insomnia, loss of appetite, and drinking too much. But I use the term in a broader way to include what people automatically find themselves doing when they are unable to get across leading-edge feelings. Such symptoms include:

1. Substitute efforts to get them across.
2. Negative feelings (e.g., frustration, boredom, hostility, and irritation resulting from a failure to get them across).
3. Attempts to deal with these negative feelings (e.g., withdrawing, becoming numb or apathetic, going to a movie as a distraction).
4. Self-blame for any of the above.
5. Attempts to relieve this self-blame (e.g., self-justification, blaming others).

I want to convince you that this is a useful way to think of symptoms.

Here is what Paul might say if, at this moment, he *were* able to put in words his leading-edge feeling:

> I'm having a hard time tonight, because instead of feeling good about you, I just feel pressured. And I worry what that means about you—and what it means about me. I go back and forth between thinking that there's something wrong with you for pressuring me and thinking that there's something wrong with me for feeling pressured. I feel like a failure as a husband. I know you're having a hard time making dinner, and I feel bad about not helping you, but your "Damn—it's completely ruined!" just felt like another pressure.

"Not hearing" Marie's exclamation—that is, continuing to watch TV—is what Paul is left to do because he is unable to get this across. At the same time, it is a substitute way for getting it across. Paul's ignoring Marie's implicit request that he come and help her is *his* implicit—that is, substitute—way of indicating that it is more than he feels he can deal with at the moment. It is Symptom 1.

But Paul is affected by Marie's outcry from the kitchen—even though he does not appear to respond to it. He finds himself bored with the News (Symptom 2). His inability to tell Marie his leading-edge feeling— that he feels bad about not coming into the kitchen to help her—further deprives him of the sense of contentment he would need to be able to kick back and pay attention to the News. Feeling bored by the News is one of the ways in which he experiences the alienation, demoralization, and loss of good feeling resulting from this disagreeable interchange in which Marie has made a nonverbal request and he has made a nonverbal refusal. At the moment, nothing looks good to Paul; nothing interests him.

He reaches for the paper in an attempt to jump-start himself into a "sense-of-contentment, able-to-relax" *un*alienated state (Symptom 3). But he finds the paper just as boring as the TV (Symptom 4). He wonders what the kids are up to (Symptom 5); just their presence often cheers him up. But then he remembers that Jeannie is playing with the little girl next door and Billy is doing his homework. Paul hopes they're doing better than he is.

So Paul goes back to the TV (Symptom 6) and impatiently switches channels, trying to find something at least a *little* interesting to watch (Symptom 7). (Of course, switching channels is not always a symptomatic act. In fact, for some people, *not* switching channels, just watching *one* show, may be symptomatic—that is, what they do when they feel dispirited.)

The result of this channel switching and overall restlessness is a *new* leading-edge feeling that Paul needs to get across in order to stop generating symptoms. He needs to be able to tell Marie (or himself):

> I went into the living room hoping to recover from the day, but I just sat there feeling bad about what happened between us when I got home. Your calling out from the kitchen was the last straw. I hated it *and* I felt bad about hating it and about not responding to it. I felt I should have come into the kitchen to help you out. So I've been in here searching through the paper and switching channels, looking for something that's capable of distracting me from all these awful feelings.

Saying this, Paul would be bringing Marie in on his alienated state. He would be shifting from the "searching-through-the-paper, switching-channels, feeling-gloomy" alienated state to the *"confiding-in-Marie*-about-searching-the-paper, switching-channels, feeling-gloomy" *intimate* state. He would be getting across what he needs to in order to stop generating symptoms.

At any given moment there is a leading-edge feeling that we all need to get across in order to avoid generating symptoms. Getting it across is what intimacy is. Not getting it across is what alienation is. And the pattern of alienation that is created by not getting it across leads to psychopathology.

Skeptic: There's a feeling that *I* need to get across to you, or *I'm* going to start generating symptoms. I'm just astonished at what you're saying. Being bored with what's on TV and turning it off isn't pathological, it's normal. Everyone does it all the time. In fact, it's *healthy* to get bored with TV; most of us watch too much of it anyway. I don't want you to take the normal things that everyone does every day—that *I* do every day—and tell me they're *abnormal*.

Wile: Well, in using the word "symptom," I'm following in Freud's footsteps. Freud (1901/1960) described as "symptomatic acts" such things as forgetting names or making Freudian slips. He saw these as normal everyday events, and in fact labeled them "the psychopathology of everyday life." I'm saying that the major psychopathology of everyday life consists of the subtle, everyday ways that everyone continually becomes alienated—from themselves and from one another. That's a main outcome of this fine-grained look at Marie and Paul's evening: discovering how they—and by extension all of us—continually go in and out of alienated states.

CHAPTER 22

Life as the Continual
Generation of Symptoms

I f you look at the moment-to-moment events of your life, you will see a succession of symptomatic acts.

While Marie is in the kitchen making dinner, Paul is watching TV generating symptoms. He:

- Ignores her "Damn—it's completely ruined!" (Symptom 1).
- Becomes bored with the TV (Symptom 2).
- Tries to absorb himself in the paper (Symptom 3).
- Wearies of the paper (Symptom 4).
- Wonders what the kids are up to (Symptom 5).
- Shifts back to the TV (Symptom 6).
- Where he restlessly switches channels (Symptom 7).

What Marie would like Paul to do, of course, is to come into the kitchen and say, "I heard you yelling. Is something wrong? Do you need any help?"

Warmed by Paul's offer, Marie might finally be able to confide, "I need a *lot* of help—with everything. Nothing's going right today."

Which, in turn, might enable Paul to confide in her, "Or *tonight*, either. We really got off on the wrong foot, didn't we?"

And Marie would nod. "We really did."

Which would immediately get them back on the *right* foot.

But none of this can possibly happen. To start with, for Paul to come into the kitchen and offer his help, he would have to be in a "concerned-about-Marie, wanting-to-help-her" state rather than his current "feeling-invaded-by-her, needing-to-keep-my-distance" state.

And for Marie to respond, "I need a *lot* of help—with everything; nothing's going right today," she would have to be in a "self-sympathetic, feeling-that-I-*deserve*-to-be-helped" state. Instead, she is in the "self-blaming, feeling-I-*don't*-deserve-anything" state.

And for Paul to respond, "We really got off on the wrong foot, didn't we?", he would have to be in a "it's-not-your-fault, it's-not-my-fault, it's-just-one-of-those-things-that-happened" state of mind rather than his current "it's-my-fault, or, if-not, then-it's-your-fault" state.

There is no way for Marie and Paul to have this conversation—neither is in the right state of mind. And that is too bad, because without such a conversation, they will continue to generate symptoms, as Paul does all through dinner:

- He has little to say (Symptom 8).
- Except to complain that the salmon is a little overdone (Symptom 9).
- And to snap at Billy for whining and at Jeannie for playing with her food (Symptom 10).

And now there is a new leading-edge feeling that *Marie* needs to get across. She needs to say to Paul (or to herself):

> I'm having a hard time. I tell myself that I should be tolerant and understanding when you're being quiet and irritable like this. After all, there are plenty of times that *I'm* quiet and irritable. So I think I *shouldn't* be upset. And I think I *shouldn't* take it personally. And I think I *shouldn't* feel lonely and resentful. But I *am* upset. And I can't possibly take it more personally. And I *do* feel lonely and resentful. I keep thinking it's because there's something wrong with me—that I'm weak and needy. So I'm sitting here feeling upset with myself for being upset with you.

In getting all this out, Marie would be appealing to Paul as an ally in helping her deal with having lost herself as one. But *how* is she going to get all of this out? Or any of it? That is the problem. It is too hard to figure out and say much of what we need to. It requires being in a different state of mind from the one we are in. It requires articulateness, wisdom, and a cool head. And these are not attributes we generally have when we have lost ourselves as an ally.

So Marie does what people typically do when they are unable to get across what they need to get across: She generates symptoms.

- She feels lonely without knowing why (Symptom 1 for her). She dimly senses that her loneliness is in response to Paul's withdrawal and irritability, but her tendency to blame herself for being needy prevents her from seeing his part clearly. Paul obviously has had a bad day, she tells herself; she should be understanding and leave him alone.

- But, feeling lonely, Marie has an urge for a hug (Symptom 2).
- She suppresses this urge immediately and reproaches herself for having it (Symptom 3).

This is what Marie is unable to tell herself:

Of course I want a hug—I need the reassurance. Paul's withdrawal and irritability are hard to take on top of a day like this, when everything's gone wrong. I need a *big* hug. And I need it even if he isn't in the mood to give me one.

Of course, in sympathizing with herself this way, she would be giving *herself* a hug—and a big one. Instead of sympathizing with herself, however, she tells herself:

Won't I ever grow up? Only children need to be hugged and pampered after every little setback. I hate myself for being so dependent and wimpy that I can't get through the day without leaning on Paul. I shouldn't be so weak and neurotic.

And then she tells herself:

Wait a minute. What's so terrible about wanting some affection from your husband once in a while? There's nothing wrong with me for wanting a hug; there's something wrong with *Paul* for being unwilling to give me one. He must be afraid of intimacy.

Marie has rescued herself from self-blame by blaming Paul (Symptom 4). But that immediately exposes her to Symptom 5: discouragement about the relationship. She tells herself:

I want hugs and Paul doesn't want to give them. I want closeness—after all, that's what people get married for—and Paul's *afraid* of closeness. We're incompatible.

Marie has passed through a common three-part sequence:

Part 1. Assassinating her own character: She is defective (Symptom 3).

Part 2. Which she defends against by assassinating her partner's character: Paul is defective (Symptom 4).

Part 3.   Which leaves her with a defective partner and a feeling of
hopelessness about their relationship (Symptom 5).

As a result of all this, Marie now has an even greater need for reassurance (Symptom 6) and an even greater need to feel close to Paul. She
suggests that they rent a video and watch it together after the kids go to
bed (Symptom 7).
But Paul says:

> They're always out of the good ones. Besides, it's raining. And I don't
> want to go out—I haven't seen the kids all day and I want to spend
> some time with them. Anyway, I don't feel like a movie.

Marie wants a hug, but she will make do with a video, and she
doesn't even get that—although she is glad that Paul wants to be with
Jeannie and Billy.
So she gives up on Paul (Symptom 8), and when he goes upstairs
to the children's room, she picks up a novel (Symptom 9). She wants to
divert herself. It's about two passionate and devoted lovers. She imagines how wonderful it would be to have a husband so totally involved
in her—and she feels better. But then she remembers the husband she
has—and she feels worse.
So Marie puts down the book and, in an attempt to do something
constructive—to get the sense of accomplishment that can come from
getting something done—she straightens her desk (Symptom 10). Marie
had been putting off straightening her desk for weeks, but now she *feels*
like doing it. Becoming symptomatic can sometimes get you enthusias-
tically tackling the very things you have been avoiding.
Having neatly arranged the bills and the outgoing mail, and still in
need of a friendly voice, Marie calls her friend Nancy (Symptom 11).
Calling Nancy is not *always* a symptom, of course, but it is for Marie at
the moment. And then, after making sure Paul has put the kids to bed
(at least she feels close to *them*, she tells herself), she writes to her sister
(Symptom 12).
Marie feels a little better—a little more connected to people—but it
is not the same as talking with Paul. So when he comes back downstairs,
she takes a deep breath and makes another attempt (Symptom 13):

> You're so quiet tonight.

Marie is trying to start a conversation in order to make things better between them. It never gets off the ground, however. Marie's "You're

so quiet tonight" is a *veiled* complaint. It is Symptom 14. She is suggesting that Paul should *not* be quiet.

And that puts Paul in a position in which he needs to be able to say:

> I know you're trying to be helpful—and I think I should be appreciating it—but I'm *not* appreciating it. For some reason your telling me I'm quiet hits me wrong.

But Paul cannot say that. All he can say is this:

> I'm just tired, that's all.

Which is Symptom 11 for him. He hopes Marie will take the hint that he doesn't want to talk about it.

And she does take it. She glances at him blankly for a second and goes into the other room. Immediately there is a new leading-edge feeling that Paul needs to get across:

> I'm glad you got the idea and left me alone. But—and I know this is a total contradiction—I'm also *sorry*. I was *disappointed* you left. I know that's got to surprise you—it surprises me. I guess it means there was something I wanted to happen between us tonight—I just don't know what it is—and your walking away meant that it *wasn't* going to happen.

Now, there is *no* way that Paul is going to be able to get that out—or even begin to formulate it. And that is too bad, because his alternative is to continue to generate symptoms, which is what he does:

- He has the flashing thought: "Women just don't understand" (Symptom 12).
- Followed by a "hollow-longing-empty" feeling (Symptom 13).
- Which he misreads as an emptiness in his stomach—hunger (Symptom 14).
- So he goes to the refrigerator and stares into it, looking for something at least a *little* interesting to eat (Symptom 15).
- And he finds nothing (Symptom 16)—or *almost* nothing. The popovers look good, but they're supposed to be for the kids' lunch tomorrow—in fact, he'd gotten them as a special treat for them.
- And suddenly he feels really tired (Symptom 17).
- He thinks it's because of work. That is Symptom 18—thinking it's only *work* that has worn him out.

• Saying nothing (Symptom 19)—in fact, acting as if Marie were not there—he goes to bed an hour earlier than usual (symptom 20).

Now Marie *really* feels abandoned. And finally she feels at least a little entitled to a complaint: It's not everybody's husband who goes to bed unexpectedly without even saying good night.

But Marie does not feel entitled enough to wake Paul. So, instead, she contents herself with washing the dishes in a noisier manner than usual, half hoping it will wake him (Symptom 15).

When Marie goes to bed, she is so upset that she cannot sleep (Symptom 16).

The evening is over. Marie and Paul have spent it generating symptoms. I shall use the total set of symptoms—the 20 I have listed for Paul and the 16 for Marie—to sort them into types. As I have defined them, symptoms are *consequences* of a person's inability to get across (to formulate and to express) leading-edge feelings.

• *Symptom Type 1: Negative feelings.*

Paul's inability to get across his leading-edge feelings leaves him feeling bored, irritable, empty, hungry, tired, and disengaged. He is quiet during dinner; later, he goes to bed without saying good night.

Marie's inability to get across her leading-edge feelings leaves her lonely, discouraged, and too upset and angry to sleep. These negative feelings become the *next* leading-edge feeling that Marie needs to get across.

• *Symptom Type 2: Attempts to deal with these negative feelings (by engaging in compensatory activities or turning attention to something else).*

Paul tries to deal with feeling bored by searching the paper and switching channels to find something at least a little interesting. He later tries to deal with feeling empty by rummaging in the refrigerator for something to fill him up.

Marie tries to deal with feeling lonely by thinking about asking for a hug and by suggesting to Paul that they watch a video together. Later, she gives up on Paul and instead reads a novel, straightens her desk, talks to Nancy, and writes to her sister.

• *Symptom Type 3: Self-blame for any of these other symptoms.*
Marie thinks, "I shouldn't be so weak and neurotic [for needing a hug]."

• *Symptom Type 4: Ways of dealing with this self-blame.*
Justifying. "Wait a minute. What's so terrible about wanting some affection from your husband once in a while?"

Accusing the other person. "There's nothing wrong with me for wanting a hug; there's something wrong with Paul for being unwilling to give me one. He must be afraid of intimacy."

- *Symptom Type 5: Substitute efforts to get across the point or feeling.*

Marie's calling out from the kitchen, "Damn—it's completely ruined!" is a substitute effort to get across this message: "I feel all alone in here and I'd really love it if you'd come in, talk to me, and give me a hand."

Paul's *not* responding to Marie's "Damn—it's completely ruined!" is a substitute effort to get across this message: "I'm not up to dealing with you at the moment."

Marie's washing the dishes with a noticeable clanking and banging is a substitute effort to get across this message: "I'm angry about your being withdrawn and irritable all evening and then going to bed early without so much as saying good night."

- *Symptom Type 6: Fantasizing*

Fantasizing is an attempt to overcome the frustrated, stuck, and helpless feeling that comes from being unable to get your point across. This is a subtype of Symptom Type 2 ("engaging in compensatory activities").

Reading the romantic novel allows Marie to fantasize about having a husband who is intimate and romantic.

Skeptic: Wait! Marie and Paul shouldn't be churning out symptom after symptom like that. There's *clearly* something wrong with them.

Wile: If so, there's clearly something wrong with *all* of us, since we *all* continually churn out symptoms.

Skeptic: Well, *I* don't. When I want a hug from my husband, I don't sit around mooning about it. I go over and give *him* a hug. I'm not like Marie; I take responsibility for my feelings. And that part about the video! If my husband didn't want to watch one with me, I wouldn't let that stop me. I'd go out and get one for myself. In fact, that's what I did a couple of days ago. As soon as I walked in the door with it, he decided he wanted to watch it after all. That was okay—I'd originally wanted to see it with him, anyway. But I *did* mind when I came downstairs half an hour later, after getting the kids to bed, and found him plopped in the chair I was going to sit in, and already watching it. So I tell him, "You couldn't wait *10 minutes*; you only think of yourself." "I was saving you the bother of having to sit through the previews and titles," he says. Can you imagine? It was *way* past the titles, so I tell him, "Yes, and apparently you're also saving me the bother of having to watch the first half of the movie." So I ask him—well, maybe not too politely—to get out of my chair, and I push the rewind button, and start the tape from the beginning: previews, titles, and all. I wasn't going to take that from him. And he gives me his "long-suffering" look—I hate that look. So when he fell asleep halfway through the movie—he always does this—I didn't wake him. I just left him there. And the next morning, he gets up all stiff from spending the night on the couch and asks me how the movie ended. But I wouldn't tell him.

Wile: Well, those sound like symptoms to *me*: letting your husband sleep on the couch, and refusing to tell him how the movie ended.

Skeptic: But he deserved it. How would you like it if you took the trouble to go out and rent a movie, and your wife started watching it before you were ready?

Wile: I *wouldn't* like it—and I'd generate symptoms too. That's my point: Everyone's continually generating symptoms—because it's impossible to get across what you need to all the time.

Skeptic: But that's what I've been saying—I did get it across. I told him he was totally selfish. And I *did* something about it. I kicked him out of my chair, and then I rewound the tape. So I *really* got it across.

Wile: Well, you got across your outrage—clearly and directly. A lot of people wouldn't be able to do that. You got it across *so* well—you seemed to say exactly what you were feeling—that it is easy to miss that there might be some softer feelings that you *weren't* getting across: how you felt *ignored*, for example, since you were the one who got the video and your husband didn't even wait for you; how you felt *hurt*, since he didn't seem to be thinking of your needs at all; how you felt *baffled*, since you couldn't understand how anyone could act this way; how you felt *lonely*, since he started watching the movie as if you weren't even there in the house; or how you felt *self-critical*, worrying, perhaps, that there's something you do that pulls for such behavior.

Skeptic: It wasn't any of those things. If I felt anything, it was *disappointed*, since this wasn't how I wanted things to go—and, well, maybe *scared*. Could I really depend on a person who seems so unconcerned about my needs?

Wile: Well then, *those* are the "soft-underbelly" feelings you needed to get across.

Skeptic: But how could I have gotten them across? I didn't even know until this minute that I was having them.

Wile: Right! That's what I'm saying. It's impossible to get across everything you need to. For one thing, as you just said, you don't always know what it is.

Skeptic: But even if I got it across, it still wouldn't do any good. My husband would simply have given me a double dose of his "long-suffering, why-do-you-have-to-be-such-a-troublemaker" look.

Wile: Of course, that would mean that you *hadn't* gotten it across—since getting it across means feeling that the other person is taking it in. And if your husband gives you his "long-suffering" look, that means that he's *not* taking it in—he's reacting against it. And immediately, you'd have something new to get across—how you felt about that look.

Skeptic: But I *got* that across. I told him to wipe his "I'm-innocent, who-me?" expression off his face. But that didn't do any good either; he just tuned me out completely.

Wile: Well, you were *criticizing* him—which is okay, except at the moment I'm talking about getting across your "soft-underbelly" feelings so you don't become symptomatic. It means getting across how you felt disappointed, scared, and cut off.

Skeptic: Sorry, but I don't buy that. I shouldn't *need* to get those feelings across. It's codependent to have to talk to others to feel better. I should take responsibility for my feelings. They're my problem, and *I* should learn to handle them on my own.

Wile: Ah—but getting across how you feel is my idea of *how* to handle them on your own. It's doing what's necessary to remain nonsymptomatic.

Skeptic: But why does it always have to be me who's doing the getting across? Why can't *he* express his feelings once in a while?

Wile: That's how *he* can remain nonsymptomatic. But at the moment we're talking about *you*.

Skeptic: I just can't imagine telling him that I feel disappointed, scared, and cut off. That's not how I talk. That's not how I *think*.

Wile: Well, right! Much of what we need to say is not how we usually talk—or even think; it feels awkward and alien. As a result, we continually generate symptoms. In fact, you're probably doing it now.

Skeptic: What are you talking about? I'm sitting here minding my own business, reading your book. How could I be generating symptoms?

Wile: I notice that you've been writing in the margins comments like "Who says?", "Nonsense," "Sexist pig," "Get to the point," and "Get a *different* point." *Those* are symptoms. Those are the kind of exasperated reactions that readers have because they can't talk directly to the author about their reactions to the book.

Skeptic (*embarrassed*): You weren't supposed to see those comments.

Wile: And there's a half-eaten bag of cheese nachos on the table. Eating cheese nachos can be a symptom too. If what you're reading produces an "empty, deprived, not-being-given-enough" feeling and, if you don't have a way to say something about it, you could get hungry.

Skeptic: Maybe I just missed lunch.

Wile: Maybe you did. Did you?

Skeptic: Well, maybe I didn't—but why should that matter? Let's say your book did make me hungry. Is that such a big deal?

Wile: It *isn't* a big deal. That's what I'm saying. It's what happens all the time. It's easy, when reading a book, to become hungry, sleepy, or bored and then to deal with these feelings by getting a snack, taking a nap, skimming the book—or, for that matter, putting the book down, turning on the TV, or starting to write your *own* book.

Skeptic: Are you saying I shouldn't be doing those things?

Wile: I'm saying you're *going* to be doing those things—or similar things. And so am I. If you have a leading-edge feeling that you can't get across, it's got to affect you in some way. You're going to become symptomatic. In fact, that's why I invented you: to give my readers a chance, through you, to get across reactions and reservations so they won't become symptomatic.

Skeptic: I don't think I like that. I thought we had a relationship—but you're saying you created me just to keep your readers from getting symptomatic.

Wile: But that's what *any* relationship is: a way to keep from becoming symptomatic. It provides the possibility of getting across something to someone when you're having trouble getting it across to yourself.

Skeptic: Now *that* sounds really interesting. Why didn't you tell me about that in the first place?

Wile: I'll tell you about it in the next chapter.

CHAPTER 23

Relationships as Solutions That Create New Problems

A relationship is a way of dealing with symptoms and, at the same time, a source of new symptoms.

As I have just described, Paul goes to bed early. From his bed, he hears Marie banging dishes in the kitchen. He realizes that she is upset—probably with him. So when she comes to bed a little later, he pretends to be asleep. He doesn't want to get into a long discussion—he has a big day tomorrow. (Of course, he wouldn't want to get into a long discussion even if he *didn't* have a big day tomorrow.)

Marie climbs into bed, tosses and turns, and adjusts and readjusts her pillow. She gets out of bed, finds another pillow, and plops back into bed, where she tosses and turns some more. She gets out of bed again. Paul hears her rustling around in the kitchen; he assumes she is getting something to eat. A little later she climbs back into bed, shaking it a little more than necessary.

Paul is in bed with a symptom-generating machine.

Of course, so is Marie. The only reason Paul knows that Marie is having trouble sleeping is that he is having trouble too. That is one of Paul's symptoms. Another is pretending that he is *not* having trouble—that he *is* asleep—which is the latest in a chain of symptoms that stretch back at least as far as Paul's inability, when he first came home, to tell Marie about his daydream that she comfort him after his bad day.

In fact, that daydream is *itself* a symptom. It is the result of an inability to get across what he has needed to say the whole day. Let us go back in time and review Paul's experiences during the day:

- Paul has to sit and take it while his boss chews him out for her mistake. She would give him only stockroom work for the next 2 weeks if he were to point out that *she*, not *he*, cleared the ad for Brontosaurus Earmuffs without checking whether they had any in inventory.

- Paul has to fake interest while the store owner tells his most boring "how-to-get-the-best-deal" story for the zillionth time.
- Paul has to bite his tongue while a customer obsesses over whether to buy a 10-cent screw. He doesn't have the satisfaction of saying, "Listen, buddy, do me a favor next time and do your shopping across the street."
- Paul has to comfort the stock clerk about mislabeling 70 cartons of Christmas decorations. The clerk is too upset about his mistake to tolerate any criticism.
- Paul has to congratulate Stanley on his promotion. It would be inappropriate to say, "How does a jerk like you get promoted when I don't?"
- Paul is *going* to tell off the bus driver for closing the door in his face, but by the time he opens his mouth, the driver is down the street and gaining speed.

Standing on the corner waiting for the next bus, Paul takes mental revenge on everyone.

Paul's 12-Second Mental Revenge

Paul imagines the bus driver crashing into a light pole, totaling the bus, and losing his job. He imagines Stanley making such a fool of himself in his new position that the owner demotes him, admitting that he should have promoted Paul, and makes Paul his special assistant—Paul is not only Stanley's boss now, but his boss's boss. And the first thing Paul does is call his former boss in and make her admit that *she* was responsible for the earmuffs fiasco.

Imagining all these things, Paul feels better—until he snaps out of it. And then he feels worse, because none of it is real. And suddenly he feels all alone—like that time as a kid when he was chased by a bully and there was no one he could tell; he didn't want to go running home to Mommy. Once again there is nobody to tell. Marie would be the natural one—but that is too much like running home to Mommy. Immediately Paul snaps into a daydream of Marie comforting him.

Paul's 12-Second "Being-Wonderfully-Comforted" Daydream

Since Paul cannot go home and tell Marie that he has had a horrible day, he has the wish that she somehow guesses it and, even now, is making preparations to cheer him up. She stops at the market to get the ingredients for his favorite meal. When she gets home, she tells the kids that their father has had a difficult day and they should go easy on him. And the kids decide to greet him at the door with that cute little duet they do that always makes him feel good. Marie is wearing the blue dress he loves; she is warm and welcoming, upbeat but not overwhelming—and beautiful. She is Earth Mother and Sex Goddess combined.

And, imagining all this, Paul feels better—until, again, he snaps out of it and realizes that none of it is going to happen. Suddenly he feels gypped. And then he feels like a heel. He says to himself:

> Expecting Marie to do all these things for me is *still* running home to Mommy. And it's totally unrealistic. How can I expect her to guess that I've had a horrible day? And even if she *were* to guess, it's not fair—wanting her to drop everything just to mother me. She's already a mother. How selfish can I get? And wanting her to get all dolled up for me? That's so sexist, it's embarrassing.

The Skeptic Objects

Skeptic: Well, I'm glad Paul realizes it. He *is* being unrealistic, selfish, and sexist.

Wile: Well, maybe—but only in his *fantasy*.

Skeptic: What's the difference?

Wile: Well, that's what a fantasy is—unrealistic. It's a license to be selfish, childish, sexist, and mean. If you can't be all these things in your fantasies, where can you be?

Skeptic: Nowhere. And Paul agrees with me that he shouldn't be having this fantasy.

Wile: But that's the problem: thinking he shouldn't have it. If he were to feel it's *okay* to have, he might be able to tell Marie about it.

Skeptic: She'd just laugh in his face.

Wile: Well, she might—*and*, at the same, secretly blame herself for not fulfilling it.

Skeptic: Yes, right! So what's the point?

Wile: Well, let's say that Paul were to tell her *right at the start* that he knows his fantasy is ridiculous. She might be able to see that he *doesn't* expect her to fulfill it.

Skeptic: But she'd probably just tell him that she's had a horrible day too and needs comforting herself; she hasn't had time to work up a good fantasy. So there they'd be—recognizing that both need comforting but that neither is in any condition to do anything about it.

Wile: Actually, there is something they could do: They could *com-*

miserate with each other—which in itself could be comforting. Each would finally have an ally, a confidant, after a day in which the major problem for each has been *not* having an ally or confidant.

Skeptic: But Paul wouldn't be getting his fantasy fulfilled. He wouldn't be getting his favorite meal or hearing the kids' little duet, and Marie wouldn't be Earth Mother and Sex Goddess combined.

Wile: But Paul might not need all of that—or even *any* of it. Just a little comfort might do it: The chance to tell Marie about the awful day he's had, the mutual commiserating, might be worth a megaton of fantasy-comforting. And, because it wouldn' be just a fantasy, he wouldn't have to snap out of it and feel awful because it wasn't true.

Skeptic: But "commiserating" seems such a pale substitute for being married to an Earth Mother or Sex Goddess.

Wile: I'm not knocking Earth Mothers and Sex Goddesses, but it misses what Paul *really* wants, which is to be able to confide in Marie about his horrible day—to have her as an ally and a confidant. In fact, Paul snaps into the Sex Goddess and Earth Mother daydream because he thinks he *can't* confide in her about his day. It seems to him too much like "running to Mommy." So he imagines Marie as these mythic characters so that he won't have to ask her for anything. Earth Mothers and Sex Goddesses are *created* to give without being asked—it's what they do for a living. But that means, of course, that Paul won't get to have her as a confidant. He won't get to tell her what a horrible day he's had. The daydream sounds good, but it misses the mark. *It* is a pale substitute.

Skeptic: What would *hit* the mark?

Wile: Well, let's say that Paul were to feel that it *is* okay to ask for things—so much so that on his arrival home, he could say:

> Hey, where are the trumpets? There was supposed to be a brass band to cheer me up after the kind of day I just had.

Paul's request for trumpets would be so clearly ridiculous that Marie would be unlikely to worry about failing him by not fulfilling it. She would be free to sympathize. She might say:

> Oh, poor baby—tell me what happened.

After the cold, depleting day Paul has just had, he would feel nourished by her concern. He might say:

> It was one thing after another. I can't remember when I felt so frustrated and powerless.

Paul would not have known before that he felt frustrated and powerless. Now he would. These feelings would have to pop out of his mouth before they could pop into his mind. And all it would take would be a sympathetic comment from Marie. He would snap into a new state of mind in which it is possible to notice these feelings—the "sympathizing-with-myself-because-Marie-has-just-sympathized-with-me" state of mind.

So Paul does not have to have his favorite meal, the kids do not have to sing their duet, and Marie does not have to transform herself into Earth Mother and Sex Goddess. All he needs is a sympathetic ear:

- To snap him into a better frame of mind.
- To allow him finally to begin to get across what he has been unable to get across to anyone (including himself) the whole day.
- To instantly transform Marie into a confidant—someone who he feels is on his side and with whom he can recover from the frustrations of the day and celebrate whatever successes he can manage to find.
- To discover the feelings that have been plaguing him all day, but that he does not even know he has.

So relationships can help you solve the problems of the day. They are opportunities to get across the leading-edge feelings that have been accumulating since you left home in the morning. They can provide you with a confidant, snap you into a better frame of mind, and help you discover feelings that you did not know you had.

Unfortunately, relationships do not always do this. Instead of helping solve problems, they often create new ones. The fact that Paul has a partner to go home to means, by the time that he gets home, he now has a *new* feeling he is unable to get across—the fantasy of being comforted by that partner. A relationship is a way of dealing with symptoms and, at the same time, a source of new symptoms. After spending all day generating symptoms because he has been unable to get across what he needs to at work, Paul spends the evening generating symptoms because he is unable to get across what he needs to at home.

Skeptic: I know I've said this before, but I still think Paul shouldn't need Marie to solve his problems; he should be able to solve them himself.

Wile: But I thought I just showed that he can't always solve his problems himself. None of us can.

Skeptic: Well, why does he have to have such an unrealistic fantasy?

Wile: Because he believes, as do you, that he *should* be able to solve his problems himself; he *shouldn't* "run home to Mommy." His fantasy of Marie as Earth Mother/Sex Goddess is a consolation prize—even though that might be hard to see, because the fantasy seems so much the *grand* prize. But we have to remember that he has the fantasy only because he feels he can't tell Marie about ordinary feelings: his discouragement about how his day has gone and his wish to be comforted. In fact, telling Marie about his bad day would allow him to discover just how discouraged—how frustrated and helpless—he feels.

Skeptic: But why should he have to talk to Marie to discover what he feels?

Wile: Because he can't discover it by himself. That's why he needs to talk to Marie. Getting his point across to Marie is his *way* to get it across to himself.

Skeptic: Why is it so important to get it across to anyone?

Wile: Because that's what we discovered when we looked at Marie and Paul's evening earlier in the book: Their failure to make their points led to all their problems. Their evening got better when they began to get across their feelings. What's beginning to become clear is that life is the moment-to-moment management of feelings, and relationships are important to the extent that they affect this moment-to-moment management of feelings. That's what this whole book is about.

Skeptic: If that's what this whole book's about, why didn't you tell me earlier? Why did you wait until *now*—the 23rd chapter?

Wile: Because I just figured it out—in this conversation with you. Like Marie and Paul, I, too, often figure things out in conversations.

Skeptic: You know, it's pretty hard to read a book when you keep being told different things about what the book is really about.

Wile: It's pretty hard to *write* a book when you keep figuring out different things about what the book is really about.

Skeptic: I don't want to hear about your problems. I want to hear about how "life is the moment-to-moment management of feelings."

Wile: Well, look at it this way. We're always having certain disturbing or disorienting feelings. Paul has one when he experienced his wish to be comforted by Marie as "running to Mommy." And we need a way to manage these feelings.

Skeptic: What do you mean "manage"? What is there to manage? If certain feelings are a problem, why don't we just get rid of them?

Wile: That's a common way we try to manage them. And it can work—at least, partly. But lots of feelings insist on hanging around—or if you *are* able to suppress them, you pay a price. For instance, if you don't get the chance to mourn the death of a person who's close to you, you could grieve underneath for the rest of your life.

Skeptic: But that's such an extreme case.

Wile: Well, the same holds true for nonextreme cases, like just now when Paul banishes his wish to be comforted. It doesn't just go away quietly. It comes back in the form of a vague uneasiness that costs him an evening. Paul senses something wrong, but he can't put his finger on it. It might be a relief, in fact, if he *were* able to put his finger on it—that is, if he could discover that the dissatisfaction and restlessness plaguing him all evening are, in part, the results of his forgotten daydream. So one way to manage feelings is to get rid of them, as you say; another way is to put your finger on them—to formulate them, to get them across to yourself.

Skeptic: So what does it *take* to put your finger on your feelings? How do you do that?

Wile: Puzzling them out in your own mind might be enough—just letting your thoughts wander until they hit upon the crucial feeling. Or it might take writing them down—say, in a diary.

Skeptic: Well, isn't that what I just said? You don't need anybody; you can do it yourself.

Wile: Sometimes. But sometimes thinking or writing isn't enough either, and that's when you might need to talk to someone—say, your husband. It may not take much—just getting your feelings into the open in his presence to feel that you've gotten them across—even if he doesn't seem to be listening, and instead argues, disagrees, interrupts, gives unwanted advice, or continues to read his paper.

Skeptic: That's still doing it myself though, since he'd be *obstructing* more than helping.

Wile: Yes, and sometimes you'd need him *not* to obstruct. You'd need him to listen—to put down the paper and pay full attention. And sometimes you might want more than that. You might need to feel he's on your side—that he sympathizes, understands, and appreciates how you feel.

Skeptic: But even then I'd just be using him as a sounding board. I'd *still* be doing most of the work myself.

Wile: In that case, yes. But remember, you don't always know what your feelings *are*. You might need his help in figuring them out. You might need him to draw you out, make informed guesses, or remind you of what you've felt in similar situations.

Skeptic: Well, I do a lot more than that with my husband. I tell him what to *do* about his problems. If my husband were in Paul's position, I'd tell him that he shouldn't let his boss get to him. And if she did, he should talk to her about it. And if that doesn't help, he should go to the store owner. And if not even that helps, he should look for another job.

Wile: How does your husband usually feel when you give him such advice?

Skeptic: Well, he doesn't follow it. In fact, he usually doesn't even *listen* to it—he goes into another room and sulks. I've never understood why.

Wile: I think I know why. If your husband were like Paul and wanted you to appreciate how he felt, then he could easily take your advice to mean that you *didn't* appreciate how he felt: that you think he just mishandled the situation—that it was a simple matter and he just didn't deal with it right.

Skeptic: Well, it *was* a simple matter, and he *didn't* deal with it right. He should have told his boss straight out that the earmuff fiasco was her fault. He should have told the owner that he was dealing with a rush order and couldn't listen to the story. He should have told the customer that the store across the street had a better selection of screws. He should have told the stock clerk to shape up or ship out. He shouldn't have let Stanley's promotion bother him. And he should realize that bus drivers can be like that sometimes—they have a tough job—and he shouldn't take it personally.

Wile: But if your husband were in Paul's position, he'd already be feeling frustrated and powerless. Telling him that he mishandled one situation after another, that they should have been a piece of cake—or, at least, that's what they would have been to you—would just make him feel *more* frustrated and *more* powerless. He'd feel like a fool; he'd think he couldn't do *anything* right.

Skeptic: Well, now that you mention it, that's exactly what I feel like talking to you. You're telling me that I would have totally mishandled this situation with my husband, that it should have been *easy* to handle—or, at least, that *you* would have done a better job of it.

Wile: Hmm.

Skeptic: Now I know why my husband goes into the other room and sulks. That's what *I* feel like doing.

Wile: Hmm.

Skeptic: So you've made your point.

Wile: Well, I wish I could have made it without *violating* it—without doing to you what I criticize you for doing to your husband. I guess this is another example of how easy it is to become accusing without knowing it.

Skeptic: Here's what I *wish* you'd have said to me. I *wish* you'd said:

> Yes, when your husband comes home after a bad day, it's hard not to feel that it's your job to help him. And then it's easy to feel that you've failed when you can't figure out how to do it. And you feel even more helpless than *he* does, because at least he has the possibility of doing something about it—like talking to his boss

or the owner of the store. I know it's hard to stand by feeling helpless when someone you care about feels so defeated. You can't stand it; you *need* him to do something about it. And I know it's hard *not* to be impatient, since it does seem to you that he's too thin-skinned. And maybe it mystifies you that he doesn't like your advice—since in your judgment, at least at the moment, it would really help.

Wile: That sounds really good! I wish I *had* said all that. I'd be appreciating *your* feelings, instead of criticizing you for not appreciating your husband's feelings.

Skeptic: And now I know what I could have told my husband if he *were* in Paul's position. I could have told him:

What miserable luck that all these things had to happen on the same day: the earmuffs, the boring story, the fussy customer, the stock clerk's mistake, and Stanley's promotion. And then when you finally got out of the store and thought you could breathe, you ran into that bus driver.

Wile: Your husband couldn't possibly feel like going into another room to sulk after hearing that!

CHAPTER 24

Therapy: Helping Clients
Get Across What They Need To

In any given situation, when people are unable to get across what they need to (often because they do not know what it is), they generate symptoms. So in therapy I try to show clients what they need to get across in order to stop generating symptoms (and that is practically all I do).

Let us say that Marie and Paul come for a couples therapy session with me the day after this night in which Paul, unable to tell Marie about his daydream that she comfort him, went to bed early, leaving Marie feeling abandoned.

MARIE (*to the therapist*): Last night was awful. Paul wouldn't talk to me. But even if he had, it wouldn't have really mattered. He never talks about what's really *important*—like how he feels about anything, including our relationship. I'm *tired* of being the only one who ever talks about our problems.

PAUL: But that's just the point: Why can't you look at the good things we have? Why do you always have to talk about problems?

MARIE: Well, someone has to—and if I left it to you, we'd never get anything straightened out. Anyway, what *are* all these good things? Name *one*.

PAUL: Well, I'm not going to tell you *now*. In the mood you're in, you'll just make fun of them.

MARIE: That's an excuse. You're not telling me because you can't think of any. And you can't think of any because there *aren't* any. And there's *nothing* wrong with my mood.

PAUL: There isn't? Listen to your tone of voice—how angry it is.

MARIE: Of course I'm angry. Who wouldn't be angry whose husband stops talking to her for a whole evening and doesn't even think it's a problem—who never thinks *anything* is a problem?

PAUL: I was just tired, that's all. Maybe I was a little quiet. So what? You always make mountains out of molehills.

MARIE: That's only because you make *molehills* out of *mountains*. You're wearing blinders. You don't think we have any problems at all.

PAUL: You don't see that there's anything *good* about us at all. *You're* the one with the blinders. And you *certainly* don't see that there's anything good about *me*. You don't notice that I have a steady job, that I'm a good father, that I do more around the house than any other husband we know, and that I'm not a workaholic. I come home on time every night.

MARIE: If you're not going to talk about anything important when you come home, who *cares* if you're on time? Who cares if you come home at all?

Marie and Paul are caught in an inconclusive and frustrating argument. They are generating symptoms. Of course, how a therapist understands this argument depends on his or her psychotherapeutic theory:

If I had Farland's "back-to-childhood" theory, I would try to see how Marie and Paul were distorting the present in terms of the past. For example, I would think about how Marie might be displacing onto Paul her unresolved feelings toward her nonengaged father, and how Paul might be displacing onto Marie his unresolved feelings toward his critical mother.

If I had Bacon's "character-defects, developmental-deficits" theory, I would look to see how the heart of the problem might be Marie's demandingness and need to control, and Paul's fear of intimacy and his own need to control.

If I had Eberheart's "serves-a-purpose" theory, I would try to figure out how Marie and Paul's argument might serve an unconscious purpose: protecting against too much intimacy, perhaps, or energizing the relationship.

But I have the "people-generate-symptoms-when-unable-to-get-something-across" theory. So I look to see what Marie and Paul are suffering from being unable to get across.

I would be thinking that, whatever *else* is going on—whether Marie and Paul are acting out unresolved issues from childhood; whether they are dependent, narcissistic, or whatever—the heart of the problem is their inability to get something across. And once you have the idea that there is something a client needs to get across, it is often easy to figure out what it is. It is obvious, as I listen to Marie and Paul, what is not getting across:

> Marie is unable to get across to Paul that there are problems in the relationship that have to be talked about—that is what she keeps saying, after all.
> Paul is unable to get across to Marie that the relationship is not as bad as she seems to think—that is what *he* keeps saying.

Why are they unable to get these points across? Because what each says in the *effort* to get his or her point across just makes the other feel unheard.

> Marie needs Paul to appreciate that it is important to talk about problems. But what Paul keeps saying—that Marie refuses to see the good in the relationship—just makes her feel that he doesn't appreciate it.
> Paul needs Marie to appreciate that there is good in the relationship. But what Marie keeps saying—that Paul refuses to talk about problems—just makes him feel that she doesn't appreciate it.

So Marie and Paul are each unable to make their points. In fact, as I have been saying, that is what a fight is. Whenever partners in my office fight—whenever I fight with my *own* wife—I immediately assume that here are two people who feel frustrated because (as in the case of Marie and Paul) what each says in the *effort* to make his or her point just makes the other feel that his or her point is *not* getting across.

And there is something *else* that Marie and Paul are unable to get across:

> Marie is unable to tell Paul how *lonely* she feels being the only one who recognizes the importance of talking about their problems.
> Paul is unable to tell Marie how discouraged and defeated he feels when Marie seems so displeased with him.

Everyone's instinctive feeling while listening to Marie continually repeat "You never talk about our problems" and to Paul's "Why do you always have to look at the negative?" would be to get them to stop. That is my instinctive feeling also. They have not come to therapy to argue in the same demoralizing way they do at home. My ideal, of course, is to get them to stop in a way that helps them make their points.

That is where the "people-generate-symptoms-when-unable-to-get-something-across" principle comes in—because it directs my attention to what Marie and Paul are suffering from being unable to get across. I am thus able to say:

> The two of you have got to be feeling pretty frustrated, because, if I understand it right, Marie, you're trying to convince Paul that there are problems in the relationship that need to be talked about, and you must be feeling lonely being the only one noticing them. But you *can't* convince Paul because, if I understand it right, Paul, you're trying to convince Marie that there *aren't* any serious problems and you feel discouraged, defeated—and maybe even a failure as a husband—when you see Marie as being so critical of you and of the relationship. So neither of you can convince the other of this one crucial thing. That's a difficult, nowhere place to be, and I can understand your having a lot of trouble with it.

Instead of telling Marie and Paul to stop their fight, I am telling them *why* they cannot stop. Namely, they both have a crucial point they need to make. In the course of telling them this, I am making their points for them. And I am doing a better job of it than they did, since I am including the following important feelings and aspects that they have left out: "frustrated," "lonely," "discouraged," "defeated," "failure as a husband," "neither . . . can convince the other," and "difficult, nowhere place to be." And they enjoy what I say. They feel that they have gotten across their points, at least to me—and, through me, perhaps to each other. Each one hopes that the partner may finally be able to listen, since it is coming from me. For a moment they stop fighting.

As I said, my task at any moment in a couples therapy hour is to figure out what each partner needs to get across. My ultimate goal is to teach them *about* the "people-generate-symptoms-when-unable-to-get-something-across" principle. I want to give them the advantage of knowing that their problems are the result of an inability to get across something important.

So that is what I do when I think I *know* what the clients are unable to get across: I tell them what I think it is. But what happens when I *don't* know? To back up a little, I don't know, when I am first told at the beginning of the hour about Paul's reactions the night before (i.e., his silence, irritability, going to bed early, not saying good night, etc.), that he was suffering from an inability to confide in Marie about his fantasy that she comfort him.

In fact, when they tell me about the previous evening, I first guess something entirely different. I ask myself:

What is the feeling that, because Paul was unable to confide in Marie about it, led to his irritability, silence, and these other symptoms?

And I answer:

Well, if Paul was silent and irritable—and if he didn't say good night to Marie—it might mean that he wanted to be left alone. So the feeling he was suffering from not getting across might be thus: "On a night like this, when I've had a rough day, I'd really appreciate your understanding that I just need to be alone and your not taking my silence and grumpiness personally."

To check out whether my guess is correct, I say to Paul:

THERAPIST: Let's try to track this down. Do you remember what you were feeling on the way home from work?
PAUL: I'd had a terrible day and I wanted to get home so I could finally relax.
THERAPIST: How did you see Marie fitting into your plan to relax?
PAUL: What do you mean?

(Every question I ask is not a perfect question that gets an immediate response.)

THERAPIST (*backing up and trying again*): Well, did you see her as helping you relax? Or did you see her as getting in the way?
PAUL: Funny you should mention that, because for a moment walking up the steps, I remembered how things used to be when we were first married. Marie would meet me at the door with a smile and a cold drink—and that would take care of everything.

THERAPIST (*to himself*): So Paul was having an "*involved*-with-Marie" fantasy, and not the "wanting-to-avoid-her" fantasy I'd guessed.

THERAPIST (*to Paul*): Could that have been what you wanted last night—a smile and a cold drink?
PAUL: It's not Marie's job to make up for my bad day.
THERAPIST: Yes, but—
PAUL: For one thing, she might have had a bad day too and needed some cheering up herself.
THERAPIST: Sure, but you could still *wish* that she was in the mood to cheer you up. And you could still feel *disappointed* if she wasn't.

THERAPIST (*to himself*): It looks like Paul has the same problem Marie has. He, too, thinks that he doesn't have a right to his wishes.

PAUL: Well, if you're saying it's all right to wish for things, listen to this. I'd forgotten—it's embarrassing—but I had this totally off-the-wall wish that Marie would magically know I'd had a horrible day. (*Turning to Marie*) You'd meet me at the door with a big hug. And you'd give me a backrub. And you'd have my favorite meal in the oven—and there'd be candles and everything. I know that's ridiculous. As it turned out, you had a worse day than I had, and you might have wanted me to do some of these things for *you*.

As Paul says this, I am thinking, "Marie is going to love hearing this, since it shows that Paul was more involved with her than she'd thought."

But Marie says to Paul:

How can you expect me to fix you your favorite meal when I've been *working* all day?

Feeling as unentitled as she does to be anything less than the Perfect Wife, Marie thinks that she *should* have fulfilled Paul's fantasy. And feeling bad about not fulfilling it, she misses Paul's main point, which is that he *knows* his fantasy is unrealistic. So I remind her:

Well, that's what Paul is saying, too—that he *didn't* expect it. He thinks it's totally off the wall. He's embarrassed by his wish.

This is an example of what I do when it is not clear what a client is unable to get across: I ask questions, which is a good thing in this situation, because what Paul needs to get across turns out to be quite different from what I think.

I have come to believe that practically all you can do with clients is to figure out at any given moment what they need to get across. You can talk to your clients about whatever you want, but if it doesn't have to do with what they need to get across, they are not going to listen. And after you finish—if they *let* you finish—they are going to come back to what is bothering them, either obliquely or explicitly. Sometimes they are not sure what it is, and I may spend the entire hour trying to help them figure it out. Sometimes they do know—in fact, they keep *repeating* it—but I do not hear it (or, if it is couples therapy, their partners do not hear it).

If I do hear it, and if I am able to help them get it across, there is often no time to rest because right on its heels there may be something *new* that they, or their partners, need to get across.

Once I help Paul get across his wish of being fussed over, I immediately have to help Marie get across that she has a hard time hearing it. Even though she realizes that Paul's wish is a fantasy that he doesn't really expect her to fulfill, she *still* feels guilty for not fulfilling it.

Paul did not know before that the sharp comments Marie sometimes makes, such as her "How do you expect me to fix your favorite meal when I've been working all day?", are motivated by guilt. Hearing this, he sympathizes with her.

But just for a moment. Almost immediately Paul gets a distant look on his face and tunes us out—which means that there is now something *new* stuck in his craw.

So there is no time to rest. Just having helped Marie establish that she feels guilty about not fulfilling Paul's fantasy—and that is why she has snapped out her objections to fixing him his favorite dinner—I now have to help Paul establish that although he thinks he should not mind Marie's snapping at him (since he sees that she is doing it because she feels guilty), he *does* mind; he is really sensitive about it. With my help, he is able to say:

> I hate it when she talks to me like that. It really bothers me. And I don't know what to do, so I just give up.

That is why he stares off into space and gets distant.

Marie has always taken Paul's distant looks as meaning that he isn't interested in what she is saying and, ultimately, that he isn't interested in *her*. Although Marie doesn't like Paul's being critical of her for snapping at him, she is glad that he is at least *reacting* to her. He is not, as she has feared, simply dismissing her. She says:

> Oh, so *that's* why you get quiet—it isn't that you don't care about me, but just that you don't like being snapped at. Hmm.

She feels relieved.

But just for a moment. Almost immediately Marie begins squirming and frowning—which means that there is now something *new* that she is unable to express.

So, again, there is no time to rest. Having just helped Paul establish that he thinks he should be tolerant of Marie's snapping at him—but that he is not; it really upsets him—I now have to help Marie establish that once again she feels that attention has been diverted from her feelings to Paul's. With my help, she is able to say:

> I never get my chance; for one thing, you've all completely forgotten everything that *I* had to deal with last night.

For a moment—and as a result of my helping her make this point—Marie feels relieved.

But something seems incomplete about what I have just helped Marie say. So again there is no time to rest.

THERAPIST (*to Marie*): I wonder if you see our forgetting about what you had to deal with last night as another example of Paul and my not understanding how you feel.

MARIE: Well, maybe—although actually, I'm just glad I was able to notice that my feelings were being overlooked—*and by me too*—because most of the time I can't do that.

And now there *is* a moment to rest—Marie is tracking her own feelings.

This is the main thing I do on a moment-to-moment basis in couples therapy: track the partners' feelings—keep tabs on what is stuck in each partner's craw from moment to moment. My ultimate goal is to put at the front of the partners' minds these ideas that are at the forefront of mine:

> I want Marie and Paul to be able to view their symptoms not as a sign that something is wrong with them (or with the other person), but as indicating that there are feelings that one or the other or both need to get across.
>
> I want them to know, whenever they are in a fight—or whenever they feel alienated from each other—that there are feelings that one or both of them are suffering from being unable to get across.

And what are these leading-edge, uppermost, major-and-immediate feelings that I say people are suffering from being unable to get across? I mean "leading-edge" and "major-and-immediate" in the sense of most profound as well as nearest the surface or most superficial. I mean one person's letting the other person in on his or her deepest worries, needs, fears, and wishes:

> I mean Marie's letting Paul in on how she feels lonely, frustrated, and abandoned when she cannot get him to see that there are problems in the relationship that need to be talked about.
>
> I mean Paul's letting Marie in on how he feels blamed, hated, beaten up, and a failure as a husband when he cannot make her see that there are good things in the relationship.

And now we know what "getting across what you need to get across" really means:

It means getting your partner to appreciate what it is like to be in your shoes.

Which may include a greater appreciation on *your* part for what it is like to be in your shoes.

Which may require help *from your partner* in figuring out what it is like to be in your shoes.

CHAPTER 25

The Impossibility of Obeying the Rules of Good Communication

The rules of good communication contain valuable bits of information. It is important to know, for example:

The difference between an "I statement" and a "you statement."
The provocative effect of saying "always" or "never."
The fact that if you express multiple complaints rather than sticking to one, your partner is unlikely to be able to listen to any of them.
The counterproductive effect of interrupting.

But there is a problem. When we look closely at the rules of good communication, we discover that they represent explicit instructions *not* to do what everyone does all the time. They are attempts to correct legislatively (i.e., by making a rule) what we do instinctively:

We are told, "Make 'I statements,' not 'you statements,'" but when we are angry, we are going to make "you statements."
We are told, "Don't say 'always' or 'never,'" but when we are frustrated, we are going to say "always" or "never."
We are told, "Don't dump out stored-up complaints," but when we feel helpless and enraged, we are going to dump them out.
We are told: "Don't interrupt your partner," but when we feel so misrepresented and so misunderstood by our partners that we cannot stand it, the rule becomes irrelevant and we are *going* to interrupt.

The rules of good communication are utopian rules; no matter what we are told, when the crunch comes we are going to do what these rules tell us we shouldn't do.

Paul and Marie's whole evening as described in this part of the book would be different if Paul were able to talk about his feelings and, in particular, if he were able to tell Marie his daydream that she comfort him after his bad day. Of course, Paul couldn't possibly tell her, because he couldn't remember it.

At best he could tell her the fragment of the daydream he *could* remember. He has a vague recollection of wishing that Marie fix his favorite meal. And that might be enough to enable him to say:

What's for dinner?

Paul doesn't know that this is his way of finding out whether Marie has fixed his favorite meal. Marie replies:

Salmon.

She hasn't. Hearing what Marie *has* prepared, Paul suddenly knows what he *wishes* she had prepared:

You haven't made Beef Belvedere in ages.

Marie is not sure, but she thinks she is being criticized. So she defends herself:

I made it for you when my sister was visiting.

And an argument begins:

PAUL: That's what I mean. That was 4 months ago.
MARIE: You're wrong. She was here 3 months ago—in October.
PAUL: It was 4 months ago—I remember clearly.
MARIE: You're wrong.
PAUL: *You're* wrong.

Marie and Paul have just disobeyed the first of the utopian rules of good communication:

• **Impossible-to-Obey Communication Rule 1: Do not get side-tracked arguing about irrelevant issues.**

It is, on the face of it, irrelevant whether Marie's sister's visit was 3 or 4 months ago. Paul could easily counter Marie's argument by saying, "Well, in either case, my point is the same: It's been *a long time* since you made Beef Belvedere." He would be countering Marie's defensive remark, regaining the initiative, and returning to the issue at hand. So why doesn't he do this? Because Paul feels too provoked by Marie's defensive remark to think clearly enough to realize that he would be in a better and more powerful position were he to sidestep it. All he can think to do is beat it down.

And now we can see why the "no-sidetracking" rule is impossible to obey. Paul is not telling Marie what he would really like her to know—about his Earth Mother/Sex Goddess fantasy, which itself is a substitute for what he wants even more: to confide in her about his horrible day. He is telling her only a fragment of his fantasy—the wish that she fix his favorite meal. And he is not even telling her that: He is just trying to get her to admit that she hasn't made Beef Belvedere in a long time. Getting her agreement on this is such a sliver of what he really wants that he cannot stand being deprived of it. Paul has snapped into the "feeling-too-helpless, frustrated, and-misunderstood-to-be-able-to-give-an-inch" state of mind:

> In the state of mind Paul was in—"wanting-to-let-Marie-know-that-it's-been-a-long-time-since-she-fixed-Beef-Belvedere"—he devoted himself to trying to get this across.
> In the state of mind he is in now—"feeling-totally-misunderstood-by-Marie, feeling-helpless, good-will-completely-vanished, Marie-is-the-enemy"—Paul devotes himself to getting even.

That is what feeling misunderstood and helpless does to Paul: It drains his good will, makes Marie seem like the enemy, and makes him unable to give an inch.

In this new state of mind, everything Marie says or does seems like a lie, a manipulation, a deceit—an attempt to get away with something. In this new state of mind, everything she says becomes an issue to challenge, a place to make a stand, an opportunity for revenge.

That is why the "don't-get-sidetracked-arguing-over-irrelevant-issues" rule is impossible to obey—because when a person is in the "blaming-the-other, seeking-revenge, can't-let-anything-pass, have-to-win-every-point" state, there is no such thing as an irrelevant issue.

And both Paul and Marie are now in this state. She, too, cannot let anything pass.

MARIE: It was 3 months ago. Remember, my sister came with us to
    Marcie's birthday party—and Marcie's birthday is in October.
PAUL: Marcie's birthday is September.
MARIE: October.

PAUL: September.
MARIE: I ought to know. She's *my* friend.
PAUL: She's my friend too.
MARIE: What are you talking about? You never *see* her.
PAUL: Well, she was my friend before she was *your* friend. In fact, I was the one who introduced you. You never would have met Marcie if it hadn't been for me.
MARIE: You're crazy. I knew her *long* before I met you. I knew her when she lived in Dayton.
PAUL: Marcie never lived in Dayton.
MARIE: Yes, she did—on Wilbur Street.
PAUL: There is no Wilbur Street in Dayton.

The irrelevant issue that began it all—whether Marie's sister visited 3 months ago or 4—has been succeeded by an avalanche of "irrelevant" issues. None of these, however, seems irrelevant to Marie and Paul.

Everyone thinks that the "don't-get-sidetracked" rule should be *easy* to obey; all you need is a little maturity. All you have to do is think about it and you will immediately see that arguing about irrelevant issues is totally counterproductive. Marie and Paul seem ridiculous—unreasonable, acting like children, self-indulgent.

And the "no-sidetracking" rule *is* easy to obey—but only when it doesn't matter; that is, when you are *not* in the "totally-frustrated, don't-let-anything-pass, there's-no-such-thing-as-an-irrelevant-issue" state of mind. When it *does* matter—when you *are* in this state of mind, which, unfortunately, is the only time you really *need* this rule—it is *impossible* to obey.

MARIE: I'm telling you there *is* a Wilbur Street in Dayton and, furthermore, that Marcie lived on it. If you don't believe me, you can call her.
PAUL: If you're so sure, why don't *you* call her?
MARIE: It's because I *am* so sure that I don't need to call her.
PAUL: Well, I'm as sure as you are, so I don't need to call her either.
MARIE: If Marcie is the good friend you say she is, you can call her and go over and have *her* cook your dinner. Maybe then you'd get something you like.
PAUL: That wouldn't be hard. You never cook *anything* I like.

Paul has just disobeyed the second rule:

• **Impossible-to-Obey Communication Rule 2: Never say "always" or "never."**

In saying, "You *never* cook anything I like," Paul is exaggerating. What he really means is that when it is Marie's turn to do the shopping, she doesn't take his preferences into account *as much as he would like.*

The problem with exaggeration is that it provokes the other person; Marie is now even *less* likely to listen to Paul. Furthermore, saying "always" or "never" is not even effective as an attack. Telling Marie that she "never" cooks anything he likes gives her an easy way out. All she has to do is point to an exception, which she immediately does:

> What are you talking about? I make rice pilaf for you all the time, because I know you love it.

Paul's "never" has allowed Marie to slip out of his stranglehold—so he is immediately sorry he said it. And he doesn't even know *why* he said it. He knows about the "always–never" rule—how it is provocative and, at the same time, gives the other person an easy way out. He wonders why he keeps forgetting this rule.

That is what I am trying to explain: why we all keep forgetting this rule, and all the other communication rules. Paul forgets them because he is in the state of mind—the "wanting-revenge, feeling-totally-helpless-to-get-across-that-I'm-feeling-totally-helpless" state—in which the rules of good communication fly out the window.

> When Paul is in the "feeling-good-about-Marie, wanting-to-collaborate, wanting-to-listen-and-be-listened-to" state of mind, the rules of good communication are relevant, and he can remember them. They are pertinent to the main thing he seeks to foster: a collaborative spirit.
>
> When Paul is in the "*not*-feeling-good-about-Marie, *not*-wanting-to-collaborate, wanting-revenge" state of mind, the rules of good communication go by the board, and he *cannot* remember them. He is interested only in finding a comment with sufficient verbal bite.

That is why Paul says "always" or "never": It *has* verbal bite. Even communication skills trainers say "always" or "never" when they are angry and want to draw a little blood. The urge to use these words can be irresistible; at times nothing but an "always" or "never" will do.

So instead of "Don't say 'always' or 'never,'" I say, "You're *going* to say them, so you might as well plan for it."

But there is one way not to use provocative statements like these, and that is to report our *wish* to use them. For example, Paul could say:

I just want to tell you that this whole conversation is driving me crazy. And I've got to say that telling me to go over to Marcie's and have her cook for me finished me off. I know I might be totally off the wall, but I felt you were telling me, "Go to Marcie and good riddance." I feel like I've been kicked in the stomach, and all I can think of right now is how to kick back.

If Paul cannot *report* his wish to kick back—that is, if he cannot get across this leading-edge feeling—then he may have no choice but to make the wish a reality and say something provocative such as "always" or "never." He makes up in firepower what he loses in precision.

And Marie immediately blows a hole in his generalization. She points to an exception. She reminds him that she cooks rice pilaf for him.

The big problem when partners try to talk—the main reason their talking breaks down—is that neither partner acknowledges anything the other says. As soon as even a subtle adversarial edge creeps into the conversation, the partners mentally hunker down. They become defensive and accusing. They become unable to say what is on their minds or to listen to each other.

To show how automatically this happens—how we take it for granted and how surprised we would be if it didn't happen—here is how it might sound if, instead of becoming defensive and accusing, Marie were to listen to and acknowledge what Paul just said. Paul would be *shocked* if Marie were to reply to his "You never cook *anything* I like" by doing any of the following:

Stopping to think about it: "Hmm. I didn't know you felt that way."

Asking more about it: "Are you saying that in anger—because we're in the middle of a fight—or do you really mean it?"

Seriously considering his position: "I'd hate to think that you're right. Let's look at it. What *do* I cook for you?"

Looking for the grain of truth in what he said: "I'm not sure about the food—we'll have to talk more about that—but I think maybe I *have* been taking you for granted recently. Maybe that's what you're picking up."

Building on what Paul said rather than tearing it down: "What you said makes me worry that you feel that I don't pay attention to what you like in other ways, too."

Appreciating Paul's position: "Well that's an awful spot to be in—feeling that your wife doesn't take into account what you like to eat—and I'd hate to think it's really true."

Appreciating how Paul might feel: "Well, you must feel pretty neglected then."

Revealing "soft-underbelly" feelings of her own: "I feel bad—that I failed you, that I'm not doing my job."

Revealing the hidden self-blame that leads to her blaming of Paul: "I feel awful; I feel that I've done something terrible. And I can't stand that—so I'm on the verge of attacking you."

Telling Paul that she is glad he told her: "I don't like what you're saying—I feel it's unfair—but if that's what you *do* feel, I need to know about it. So, despite everything, I'm *glad* you told me."

When was the last time Marie said any of these things to Paul? When was the last time anyone said any of these things to anyone? We are so used to having what we say ignored, discounted, or refuted—and doing the same to others—that we take it as a matter of course. We are unaware that there is an alternative.

I have made up this list of possible responses to give a taste of what people can get from their partners, but rarely do—and have learned to do without. I want to show how deprived we all are—although we don't know it. I want to reveal the ongoing low-grade verbal abuse we only vaguely sense that we inflict on others and that others inflict on us.

Marie and Paul are caught in a vicious circle of this kind of abuse. Paul's not listening to Marie turns her into someone who cannot listen to him. In turn, Marie's not listening to Paul turns him into someone who cannot listen to her.

To interrupt this circle—to get partners to stop ignoring, discounting, and disputing what the other says and, instead, to *acknowledge* it—communication skills trainers propose the "paraphrase" or "active-listening" rule:

• **Impossible-to-Obey Communication Rule 3: Paraphrase—repeat what your partner says in your own words, then check to see if you have it right.**

Obeying the "paraphrase" rule means doing these things:

• Listening to what your partner says—rather than ignoring, discounting, or disputing it.
• Repeating it back—to prove you *are* listening.
• Repeating it back *in your own words*—to prove you are thinking about it and not just mouthing the words.

- Repeating it back *to your partner's satisfaction*—to check the accuracy of your restatements ("Do I have it right?").

Here is Marie listening to Paul's statement, "You never cook *anything* I like," and trying to paraphrase it:

So you're telling me that I shop and cook as if you didn't even have a vote in this family—that I don't take into account what you like to eat. Do I have it right?

Now, it is hard to imagine Marie's saying this. The words may well stick in her throat. The "paraphrase" rule is difficult to obey when, as is true of Marie at the moment, you are feeling too unlistened to yourself to feel even a little like listening to the other. At such a moment, it is hard even to *remember* this rule. Marie doesn't want to paraphrase what Paul says; she wants to beat it down.

Let us imagine that a communication skills trainer was standing at Marie's elbow reminding her of this rule and encouraging her to give it a try—even if the words *do* stick in her throat. What the trainer would be recommending, in essence, is that Marie behave as she would if she were in a different state of mind from the one she is in.

That is the point, at least as some communication skills trainers and behavior therapists see it. They want us to behave as if we *were* in a different mental state. A change in behavior, they believe, can lead to a change in feelings. Behaving as if she were already in a collaborative state might jump-start Marie *into* such a state.

And it might. I have said that we have only limited control over our states of mind; I have not said that we have *no* control. If Marie behaved as if she were already in a collaborative state, that might jump-start her into such state. Or it might jump-start *Paul*. Noticing Marie's effort to be nice, and appreciating that effort, *he* might snap into a collaborative state, which in turn might snap Marie into one.

But there is no live-in communication skills trainer standing at her elbow when she and Paul are fighting. Instead of responding to Paul's "You never cook *anything* I like" by paraphrasing it, she defends herself. She says, "What are you talking about? I make rice pilaf all the time, because I know you love it." And the argument continues:

PAUL: What makes you think that? I never said I liked it that much.
MARIE: Well, you'd never know it the way you wolf it down.
PAUL: I just don't want you to feel bad—I know how much time you take to make it come out right. I'm just being considerate.

MARIE: I should cherish the moment, then—because you're never considerate about anything else.

PAUL: Just how "considerate" do you think it was to get the rugs cleaned the day of my poker game? We had to play on the kitchen table.

MARIE: That was *5 years* ago. Are you going to hold that against me forever?

PAUL: Well, you did it on *purpose.*

MARIE: Why would I do it on purpose? What could I possibly get out of it?

PAUL: I don't know. Maybe you wanted to embarrass me in front of my friends.

MARIE: That's crazy. You do that just fine all by yourself. But if you really want to talk about embarrassing people in front of their friends, how do you think *I* felt when you walked into the kitchen in your underwear with Julie sitting right there?

PAUL: Oh, come on. I didn't know she was there. You didn't tell me she was coming over.

MARIE: If I could see the future I *would* have told you—but she just dropped in.

PAUL: Well, you could at least have called out from the kitchen that she was here.

MARIE: What for? It never occurred to me that you were going to parade around in your underwear.

PAUL: Parading? I'd just come out of the shower and I was looking for my watch. You're a fine one to talk—walking around all day in your dirty warmup suit.

MARIE: That's *totally* different.

PAUL: *I'll* say it is. I came into the kitchen in my underwear *once.* You've got that thing on practically every day.

MARIE: Well, call the police. I thought a person had a right to wear what she wants in her own home.

PAUL: Other people live here too—people who might not appreciate living with a slob. You're setting a fine example for Billy and Jeannie.

MARIE: You *would* bring the kids into it. I suppose you're the epitome of elegance in that tattered bathrobe you're so attached to.

PAUL: There's nothing wrong with my . . .

MARIE: Cheapskate. You won't lay out 50 bucks for a new one.

Between the two of them, Marie and Paul have just disobeyed Impossible-to-Obey Communication Rules 4 through 10.

- **Impossible-to-Obey Communication Rule 4: Stick to one topic.**

There is already more on the docket than Marie and Paul can possibly handle. It doesn't help to bring up new inflammatory topics like Marie's getting the rugs cleaned at the wrong time, Paul's walking into the kitchen in his underwear, her dirty warmup suit, and his bathrobe. So communication skills trainers have the fourth rule: "Stick to one topic."

If we look closely, however, we will see that Marie and Paul *are* sticking to one topic—an overarching one: "Your criticism of me is totally invalid, and, anyway, you do the same—or something *worse*." The specific issues they are discussing are pieces of evidence they believe will prove their points regarding this overarching topic. Marie and Paul are saying, in essence, "Your criticism of me is totally invalid, and, anyway, you do the same thing and worse, and here is Exhibit A and Exhibit B and . . ."

• **Impossible-to-Obey Communication Rule 5: No dumping out stored-up complaints.**

Marie's wearing a dirty warmup suit around the house has been bugging Paul for some time. He has kept his mouth shut up to this point because he hasn't wanted to start a fight. Furthermore, he privately agrees with Marie that she has the right to wear what she wants in her own home.

And now that Paul *has* brought it up, he has picked the absolutely worst possible time—the middle of a fight—when he and Marie have the least possibility of discussing it in any kind of useful way. Marie is too upset about what Paul has already said to listen. Since Paul is angry, he is not saying it in the best possible way. Raising it now just makes an already bad situation worse.

So communication skills trainers devised the fifth rule: "No dumping out stored-up grievances—in fact, do not store them up at all; express them as they come up." This seems a useful rule—and similar to my point, "if you don't get across your leading-edge feeling, you are going to become symptomatic."

So it is too bad that this rule is impossible to obey when you are in the only state of mind in which you really need it—the state in which you feel:

"Why make an issue of it?"
"Don't rock the boat."
"You shouldn't cause problems when you don't have to."
"If you ignore it, maybe it will go away."
"What good would it really do to talk about it? It will just hurt his (or her) feelings or start a fight."

"You shouldn't burden him (or her) with your feelings. You should take care of them yourself."

"Why bring it up and ruin the evening?"

"And, anyway, you shouldn't let it bother you so much."

"You should focus on the good things you have rather than on the bad—think of the glass as half *full*."

These are the thoughts Paul has when he is in what I call the "don't-be-so-bothered-by-it, let-sleeping-dogs-lie" state of mind—a state that everyone is in at least some of the time (many people are in it most of the time). When Paul is in this state, he is *not* going to "express complaints as they come up." For one thing, he doesn't want to wake the dogs.

So, instead of "Do not store up complaints," I say, "You are *going* to store them up—and it is important to know that." And instead of "Do not dump out these stored-up complaints," I say, "You are *going* to dump them out—and I want you to know that, too."

Of course, dumping them out is not entirely bad. If, as I say, it is inevitable that you are going to store them, you need a way to unload them. Although the middle of a fight is the *worst* time to get them out, it may be the *only* time. For example, it is only then that Paul is not concerned about the impact of his complaints on Marie—that they will hurt her feelings or start a fight. In fact, his concern at such a moment is only that his words will not have *enough* impact. And once he does dump out his complaints, they are out in the open, and he and Marie at least have the *possibility* of a useful conversation about them later on.

• **Impossible-to-Obey Communication Rule 6: No digging up grievances from the ancient past.**

Paul's complaint about Marie's having the rug cleaned on his poker day demoralizes and enrages her. She is upset that he is still angry about something that happened so long ago. She worries that he is *never* going to let her live it down.

So communication skills trainers devised the sixth rule: "Do not dig up grievances from the distant past; stick to the present."

And Paul is not even sure why he *has* dug up this old grievance. Whenever he dug it up before, Marie called him on it. She would say, just as now—"Are you going to hold that against me forever?"—which immediately made Paul sorry he even thought of it.

But it is easy to see why he does it now. Marie has just said, "I should cherish the moment, then—because you're never considerate about anything else." Smarting from this remark, Paul snaps into the "I-can't-stand-it-when-she-gets-sarcastic-like-that, I've-got-to-retaliate" state. All he cares about is proving that *she*, not he, is the inconsiderate one. He searches his mental database of recent events, looking for evidence. And he comes up blank. So he sorts through his mental file of *not*-so-recent events—and he is rewarded with the "rug-cleaning-on-my-poker-day" incident. At the moment, he does not *care* that it occurred 5 years ago; he is just happy to find something.

Of course, the next moment—when Marie accuses him of holding grudges forever—he *does* care, but by then it's too late.

So now Paul has a new problem: how to justify holding this grudge. He does so by insisting that Marie's having the rug cleaned on his poker day was not just an act of thoughtlessness; she did it on *purpose*. He figures that there is no statute of limitations for holding a grudge about something another person does with malice aforethought. At the moment, Paul does not care that he is disobeying the next rule:

• **Impossible-to-Obey Communication Rule 7: No "mind reading." Do not tell the other person what he or she is thinking, feeling, or trying to do. Do not impute motivation.**

In telling Marie that she disrupted his poker game on purpose, and that she wanted to embarrass him in front of his friends, Paul is "mind reading." He is telling her what she was trying to do. People do not like being told what they are trying to do—even when you are right, which you usually aren't. They *particularly* don't like it when (as is also usually the case) you tell them that what they are trying to do is something generally thought of as "bad"—that is, as something they *shouldn't* be doing.

The rule against mind reading is impossible to obey, however, when you are in a "back-against-the-wall, I've-got-to-find-a-way-to-justify-what-I-just-said, I-don't-care-what-it-takes" state.

Marie responds to Paul's accusation that she wanted to embarrass him in front of his friends by accusing him of embarrassing *her* in front of *her* friend, Julie, by coming into the kitchen in his underwear.

Paul snaps into the "okay, if-that's-the-way-you-want-to-play-it, if-you're-going-to-remind-me-of-something-that-I-was-embarrassed-about-already, let's-see-how-you-feel-about-my-bringing-up-something-that-*you*-won't-like" state of mind. He brings up the issue of her dirty warmup suit.

And Marie does *not* like it. So she gets sarcastic—"Well, call the police"—which infuriates Paul. So he drops his bomb. He calls her a "slob."

In so doing, Paul disobeys yet another rule:

• **Impossible-to-Obey Communication Rule 8: No labeling or name calling.**

Paul does not need a communication skills trainer to tell him not to call Marie names. He knows that doing so breeds ill will. The "no-name-calling" rule is impossible to obey, however, when Paul is in the "feeling-totally-done-in, hating-Marie, needing-to-blast-her" state of mind.

And Marie responds with a laser blast of her own. She criticizes him for wearing a tattered bathrobe and calls him a cheapskate.

In the throes of the battle, it hardly matters that Marie has just dis-obeyed the next rule:

• **Impossible-to-Obey Communication Rule 9: No interrupting; let the other person finish.**

This rule is no more possible to obey than any of the others. It is impossible to obey when you are in the "I-can't-stand-listening-any-more, I'm-feeling-too-misunderstood-and-frustrated, what-you're-saying-is-outrageous-and-totally-unfair, I've-got-to-rebut-it-right-away" state of mind.

So those are 9 of the 10 impossible-to-obey rules of communica-tion that I wish to discuss. (I will get to the final one shortly). Taken together, these 10 show how to talk so that your partner will listen and how to listen so that your partner will talk (to slightly alter the title of Faber & Mazlish's [1980/1982] book). The more effectively partners are able to talk and listen, the better they will be able to get across their leading-edge feelings, and the less likely they will be to generate symptoms.

So the rules of good communication *can* help partners remain nonsymptomatic. They are impossible to obey, however, when partners have *already* become symptomatic—which, unfortunately, is when they most need these rules. Obeying the rules of communication at such a time requires being in a different state of mind from the one they are in. It means listening when they are both in the "feeling-too-unlistened-to-myself-to-have-any-interest-in-listening" state of mind. It means not interrupting when every fiber in their bodies is pressing to interrupt. It requires responding nonsymptomatically to the partner's symptomatic response. It requires remaining unprovoked in the face of the partner's provocative response.

How would it look if Marie or Paul *were* to react nonsymptomatically to the other's symptomatic response? Pretty strange. Let us try to imag-ine it. Let us suppose:

- That Paul were *not* to become defensive when Marie pointed out that she *does* cook something he likes—rice pilaf—but, instead, were to say: "You know, I guess I felt really *hurt* when you suggested I go over to Marcie's and have her cook for me. So I got angry."
- Or that Paul were *not* to retaliate when Marie accused him of being inconsiderate, but, instead, were to say: "I hope you don't really mean that; I'd hate to think you really see me as thoughtless."
- Or that Marie were *not* to criticize Paul for digging up a grievance from the distant past, but were to say: "I can't stand your bringing up something from so long ago—but since you did, I guess it means that I upset you more than I realized."
- And that Marie were *not* to become defensive when Paul accused her of trying to embarrass him in front of his friends, but were to say: "I hope you're saying that only in the heat of the moment—because I'd hate it if you believed I'd really do such a thing."
- And that Paul were *not* to get defensive when Marie dealt with his charge about her dirty warmup suit by pointing to his tattered bathrobe, but, instead, were to say: "You know, you're right. It's a total double standard. I've got some nerve asking you to dress any better than I do."

In making these statements, Marie and Paul would be responding nonaccusingly and nondefensively to the other's accusing or defensive response. They would be replying to the other's "you statement" by making an "I statement." They would be obeying the most famous impossible-to-obey communication rule of them all:

- **Impossible-to-Obey Communication Rule 10: Make "I statements," not "you statements."**

This rule is implicit in each of the other rules. Or, to put it another way, the other rules define various types of "you statements":

"No labeling or name calling" means essentially do not make "you statements" such as "*You're* a nag," "*You're* a slob," or "*You're* a cheapskate"—that is, do not turn your partner into a caricature with *one* identifying, negative quality.

"Never say 'always' or 'never'" means essentially do not make "you statements" such as "*You* never do such-and-such" or "*You* always do such-and-such"—that is, do not leave your partner with no room to change or be different.

"No digging up grievances from the distant past" means essentially do not make accusations (e.g., "you statements") about things in the past—that is, leave room for your partner to live it down (to be forgiven).

"No 'mind reading'" often means do not make accusations (e.g., "you statements") such as *"You're* trying to make me feel guilty."

"No dumping out stored-up grievances" means essentially do not dump out stored-up accusations (e.g., "you statements")—that is, do not come at your partner with so many criticisms all at once that he or she has no possibility to defend himself or herself.

"Do not get sidetracked arguing about irrelevant issues" means essentially do not get sidetracked arguing (e.g., making "you statements") about irrelevant issues.

"Stick to one topic" often means do not defend against the other person's accusations (e.g., "you statements") by making counter-accusations (e.g., "you statements") about something completely different.

"Do not interrupt" sometimes means do not *interrupt* the other person's accusation (e.g., "you statement") with an accusation (e.g., "you statement") of your own.

"Paraphrase what your partner says" typically means resist the urge to defend yourself or to make an accusation (e.g., "you statement") and, instead, acknowledge what the other person has just said.

The "I-statements, not-you-statements" rule—and *all* the rules of good communication—are attempts to eliminate accusation and defensiveness by fiat.

Skeptic: Gee, I've always liked those rules—they seemed to make so much sense. I've been meaning for a long time to sit down and memorize them. But now, after what you just said, I probably shouldn't bother.

Wile: Well, I've also said that they *are* worth remembering—they contain crucial bits of information. My only problem with them is that they require you to pretend that you're in a "collaborating" state when you're really in an "adversarial" state.

Skeptic: Maybe it's good to pretend you're in a "collaborating" state. Maybe, as you mentioned, pretending can sometimes make it come true— it can snap you into that state.

Wile: But only maybe, and only sometimes. Most people can't do it—or they can't do it very well. They try, fail, and feel awful about it. Or they blame their partners for the difficulty—and see them as the failures.

Skeptic: Well, I hate to give up these rules. They seem like such good ones.

Wile: They *are*—as long as we take the "rule"-ishness out of them.

Skeptic: Then what would be left?

Wile: The information underlying the rule—and it's important information. It's important, for example, to know what an "I statement" is and how it differs from a "you statement." It's important to know that saying "always" or "never" is provocative. I'd like to tap these rules for what they reveal. I'd like to use them as sources of *information*, rather than as rules that have to be obeyed.

PART 7

PICTURES

I have talked earlier in the book about how the therapist, like the client, shifts into and out of alienated and unalienated states of mind. But the therapist also shifts among theories—I call them "pictures"—which I talk about now.

In Chapter 26, I describe how each therapist has his or her own set of primary, secondary, and rejected "pictures" that, taken together, constitute his or her therapeutic approach. In Chapter 27, I describe *my* "pictures," with particular emphasis on my primary ones. In Chapter 28, I describe how my goal in therapy is to get clients to adopt my primary pictures.

Primary, Secondary, and Rejected Pictures

When I do therapy, I sometimes find myself losing sight of the major principles of my approach; that is, I am unable for a period to see how these principles apply to what is happening at the moment. At such times, I react to moment-to-moment events by adopting moment-to-moment theories—*and I do not like it*. I prefer to keep the major principles of my approach continually in my mind. So I have sat down to figure out what is going on and whether there is anything I can do about it.

Let me take as an example my individual session with Marie, described in Chapters 6 through 8. A major issue in this session is Marie's "scared-little-mouse" feeling. "My mind goes blank," Marie says; ". . . it's like I'm paralyzed." She goes on to say that when she told all this to Dr. Farland, her previous therapist, Farland told her that Marie might have been sexually abused by her father.

Hearing this, I immediately think, "Sexual abuse? Let me check that out." Implicit in these words is a train of thought that brings about an immediate shift in theory. If I were to run through the complete train of thought rather than the half-second contracted version that I give in Chapter 8, it would go as follows:

Is Farland jumping to conclusions? Is she making too much of Marie's "My mind goes blank . . . it's like I'm paralyzed"?

Or was this just the latest of a *series* of signs that Farland saw as pointing to incest?

And *are* there other signs? Does Marie have problems with trust and intimacy? Is she subject to dissociative states?

Since Marie said that *Farland* thought that she was abused, does that mean that Marie herself doesn't remember it?

And if she doesn't remember it, does that mean it didn't happen? There is the danger, then, of Farland's and my confusing Marie—and blaming her father for something he did not do.

Or does it mean that it *did* happen, but that Marie cannot remember? In that case it might be my job, as it might have been Farland's, to help her remember.

If it comes out that Marie *was* sexually abused by her father, would it be helpful for her eventually to confront her father?

Of course, I would have to be careful not to talk Marie into something she does not want to do—since that would continue the abuse.

In fact, it is important *in general* to help Marie become aware of subtle (and not always so subtle) ways in which the abuse is continually being recreated in her relationships with others—which includes her relationships with Paul and with me.

Of course, Marie might prefer to deal with this whole issue with a female therapist.

And she might get a lot out of an incest survivors' group.

Freud was more correct than he knew in his pre-1897 belief that childhood trauma—and, in particular, incest—was a root problem.

Ruminating more broadly, could it be true, as I have heard speculated recently, that the cause of borderline personality disorder is childhood sexual abuse?

At the moment, I think it also *might* be true—and as I've also heard—that all adult psychopathology is one form or another of post-traumatic stress disorder.

So *this* is the new theory of therapy I snap into—although I am not fully aware of it at the time—when I tell myself, "Sexual abuse? Let me check that out."

In checking it out, I start by asking Marie whether she thinks Farland was right. Marie says that she remembers the *opposite*—that her father didn't seem very interested in her. Or her mother either, for that matter. And her mother didn't do anything about her father's ignoring her. In fact, now that she thinks of it, what she most hates about being a little mouse is that it's so weak and timid—it's the way her mother acted so much of the time.

By answering a question about her father's possible abuse by talking about her mother's being weak, Marie could be alluding to her mother's failure to protect her. In other words, the way Marie denies the possibility of abuse provides further indirect suggestion that it might have occurred. I miss the connection, however. It is only afterward, while writing my notes about the session, that it clicks into place. I miss it because I have already shifted to *another* theory. In fact, Marie's statement that she hates being weak because that was the way her mother acted so much of the time *leads* to my shift. Hearing this, I immediately think, "Okay, so Marie is trying *not* to be like her mother." Implicit in these few words is the following train of thought and the shift in theory that goes with it:

> Marie is basing her life, in part, on trying to be different from her mother—she is suppressing that part of her that *is* like her mother.
> She clearly has unfinished business with her mother.
> And Marie also has unfinished business with her father—she feels he was uninterested in her.
> And that means that whenever Paul appears uninterested in her, she will snap back 20 years and react to him as if he were her father.
> Marie's problems with Paul are the result of her unfinished business with her parents.
> In fact, that is what everyone's problems *always* are—the result of unfinished business with parents.
> So I need to remember that whenever Marie says anything about Paul or me that seems overstated or doesn't quite fit, she is probably really talking about her mother or father.

The first theory is related to the second one. A traumatic event in childhood, such as father–daughter incest for which the daughter remains amnesic, is an extreme form of unfinished business with parents. The two theories lead in different directions, however:

> Since I am thinking of unfinished business with parents in general, I am looking to see how Marie's problems with Paul reflect or repeat those she had with her parents.
> If I were thinking of incest, I would be looking more narrowly for evidence for or against incest.

"If I see myself as a timid mouse," Marie goes on to say, "it ruins me—there's no recovery. I lose every shred of self-respect." Hearing this, I immediately think, "Oh, so Marie is *ashamed* of feeling weak." Implicit in these few words is the following train of thought, which brings about still another shift in theory:

> Shame *always* plays a crucial role in problems.
> Why do I keep forgetting that?
> Good thing Marie reminded me.
> Marie's problem is not only *being* "paralyzed," "weak," and like her mother; it is *hating herself* for these behaviors.

At the root of Marie's problem are shame, guilt, humiliation, and self-hate.

Which should not be surprising, since these are at the root of *everyone's* problems.

In the course of just a few minutes, I have shifted from the "all-problems-are-essentially-post-traumatic-stress-disorder" theory to the "all-problems-are-the-result-of-unfinished-business-with-parents" theory and finally to the "all-problems-are-the-result-of-shame" theory.

In the next session, Marie reports feeling hesitant to tell Paul that it was his turn to do the vacuuming. Hearing this, I think, "Maybe the assertiveness training people are right." Implicit in these few words is the following train of thought, which brings about yet a new shift in theory:

Marie didn't assert herself with Paul—probably because she didn't want to be seen as a nag.

Marie needs a non-nagging way to tell Paul what she feels.

Greenholtz would say she needs assertiveness training. And maybe she does.

For that matter, she might also profit from communication training, problem-solving training, negotiation training, or "fair-fight" training.

From an important point of view, Greenholtz is right that having a good relationship requires mastering a set of skills.

Maybe all problems are essentially skills deficits, and therapy is essentially skills training.

Throughout any therapy session, my mind is captured by different slices of different theories—particularly at moments when I am unable to see how my own major principles apply. If, in a couples therapy session, Marie were to say that Paul drank too much the previous night, I would think, "Oh? Could Paul be an alcoholic?" Implicit in these few words is the following train of thought, leading to an immediate shift in theory:

Check for alcoholism.

You won't accomplish anything until the drinking stops.

And first the alcoholic might need to hit bottom.

Don't be one of those therapists who misses when alcoholism is the heart of the problem.

And keep in mind that Alcoholics Anonymous might be the only effective treatment.

Alcoholism is an addiction—and there are special difficulties in treating addictions.

On the other hand, some sort of addiction lies at the root of all problems.

In fact, the goal of therapy might be to discover and confront the client's particular addictions, whatever they are.

If Marie were to say that she is sensitive to Paul's drinking because her father was an alcoholic, I would quickly append to this theory the following concern about the adult child of an alcoholic:

Is Marie a coalcoholic, a codependent, an enabler?

Was she an overresponsible "adult child" who never really had a childhood?

Was she caught up as a child—is she caught up now—in keeping family secrets, trying to be inconspicuous, trying to be good?

Should I refer her to an Al-Anon or an Adult Children of Alcoholics group?

If Marie were then to say, "Things get pretty ugly sometimes when Paul drinks," immediately I would think, "Oh? Does Paul hit her?" Implied in these few words is the following train of thought, bringing about the next shift in theory:

There's always the danger of seeing a couple for a long time without realizing that the wife is being battered.

Look for subtle signs of physical abuse.

Don't be one of those therapists who go along with the partners' minimizing of the physical abuse.

Marie might be too afraid, ashamed, and self-blaming to do more than hint at it—and what Marie just said might be the hint.

It's my job to root out the battering—and in a way that doesn't put Marie at further risk.

The first priority has to be assuring the battered partner's safety.

If couples therapy doesn't immediately stop the abuse, I must find some program, treatment, or modality that will.

Work toward freeing Marie to leave Paul if he is addicted to abusing her.

And refer Paul to a group.

Marie says that what she means by "Things get pretty ugly sometimes" is Paul's calling her names. There is abuse, she is saying in essence, but it is verbal abuse.

Paul breaks in at this point and says to Marie, "Well, you've got your own problems, you know—for one thing, you're afraid to cross the Bay Bridge." Paul's comment reminds me that Marie has had debilitating phobias for years. I immediately think, "Oh, yes, Marie's phobias." Implicit in these few words is the following train of thought, which constitutes *two* distinct theory shifts:

Theory 1

Marie's phobias might play a larger role in their problems than I realized.

I might be out of my element here. I am a psychodynamic therapist, and, from what I've heard, phobias are better treated by systematic desensitization.

Marie needs to be seeing Paul Wachtel (1977), the psychodynamic therapist who feels comfortable using behavioral methods such as systematic desensitization.

Should I refer Marie for systematic desensitization? I wish Wachtel were in town so I could refer her to him.

Since systematic desensitization does seem to work, does it mean that the theory behind it is correct? Could conditioned fear be at the root of phobias?

In fact, could it be true, as some say, that conditioned fear lies at the root of all psychological problems?

Theory 2

And I might be out of my element for yet another reason: I've heard about the success in treating fear and anxiety reactions with drugs.

So should I refer Marie for evaluation for panic disorder medication?

There's even been success treating obsessive–compulsive disorders with drugs.

Could the pharmacological psychiatrists be correct that all psychological problems are the result of biochemical imbalances?

These are examples of how, in the course of a single therapy session, I shift theories. I know there are therapists who do not shift as much as I do. In fact, some therapists maintain one theory no matter what the client says or does. Let us imagine that Marie comes in for a therapy session and says that she has a bridge phobia:

A therapist totally committed to the "intrapsychic-conflict" theory would look for the buried conflict responsible for Marie's phobia. This therapist would not consider an approach like systematic desensitization.

A therapist totally committed to the "family-homeostasis, identified-patient" theory would look to see how Marie's phobia maintains the family system (Marie is the identified patient). This therapist would not consider an approach such as systematic desensitization, either.

A therapist totally committed to the "conditioned-fear" theory would not have to shift. From the beginning, he or she would be looking for phobias, which he or she believes underlie all psychological problems.

Whereas some therapists make fewer shifts in theory than I do, others make *more*. These therapists go out of their way to combine elements from a large number of theories in their belief that each theoretical approach contains a grain of the truth. They pride themselves on being catholic.

As I said at the beginning of the chapter, I do not like shifting among theories—I like to stick to the interrelated set I see as fundamental. As I also said at the beginning of the chapter, I have tried to figure out what was going on—and whether to do something about it. I have tried to understand what these theories actually are—and what I should call them. Are they "theories"? Are they "paradigms"? Are they "models," "orientations," "frameworks," "perspectives," "positions," or "stances"?

I have decided to call them "pictures."

I have chosen the word "pictures" to suggest that, in the course of a therapeutic hour, you shift among them as you might flip through snapshots in an album (although you can also hold onto a single picture throughout a whole hour—or a whole course of therapy).

I have also chosen the word to suggest that these ideas or images completely take over your mind, becoming all you can see—much as a picture in front of your eyes completely covers your field of vision.

Primary Pictures

As I see it, each therapist has his or her own set of what I call "primary pictures":

Primary pictures are the basic beliefs that you have about people. They are the theories you have in your mind most of the time: even before your clients walk into your office, even where there is no immediate evidence—even perhaps when there is *contradicting* evidence.

Let us say that the "holdover-from-childhood" picture is one of your primary pictures—which means that when you see symptomatic behavior, you automatically wonder what kind of childhood the person must have had to lead to such behavior. If you are such a therapist, you maintain the idea that what a husband says about his wife is really about his parents, even if you cannot immediately see how. You assume that the connection is there, but that you just don't have enough information to make it yet.

Or let us say that the "family-homeostasis, identified-patient" picture is one of your primary pictures—which means that when you see symptomatic behavior in a family member (the identified patient), you automatically think, "How does this behavior maintain family homeostasis?" If you are such a therapist, you hold the belief that, for example, a wife's agoraphobia maintains family homeostasis, even if you cannot immediately see how. You assume that it does, but that you just haven't figured it out yet.

If the "irrational-ideas, negative-self-talk" picture is one of your primary pictures—as it is for most cognitive-behavioral therapists—you continue to believe that beneath a client's depression is negative self-talk, even if you have not yet been able to discover what this negative self-talk is.

If the "people-generate-symptoms-when-unable-to-get-something-across" picture is one of your primary pictures—as it is for me—you maintain this picture, even if you cannot immediately see how getting something across may help or what it is that the person may *need* to get across. You just keep looking.

"Primary pictures" are ultimate explanatory principles, final explanations, the core beliefs. They are the rock-bottom ideas that, once reached, tell you that you need go no further—you are at the *heart* of the problem.

Secondary Pictures

In addition to "primary pictures," every therapist has his or her own set of "secondary pictures":

> *Secondary pictures* are *not* typically at the forefront of your mind. You do *not* have them even before the client walks into your office. You have them only when there *is* immediate evidence. And you can easily shift out of them.

Let us say that you are a couples therapist with a classical cognitive-behavioral approach—which, as I see it, means that your primary pictures are as follows:

> The "skills-deficit" picture, in which you attribute the couple's problem to skills deficits and engage in skills training.
>
> The "positive-reinforcement" picture, in which you attribute the partners' problems to their use of aversive measures to control each other's behavior (i.e., punishment and negative reinforcement), and you encourage their use of positive measures (e.g., "pleases," positive behavior exchange, and "love days" or "caring days").
>
> The "cognitive-restructuring" picture, in which you attribute the couple's problem to irrational ideas and unrealistic expectations, which you refute and challenge.

There you are, shifting among these three pictures, doing classical cognitive-behavioral couples therapy, when suddenly a client says that her anger at her husband feels like her anger at her father. Immediately you snap into the "holdover-from-childhood" picture. You engage in cross-theory leakage. For a moment you become a psychodynamic therapist. Since the "holdover-from-childhood" view is only a secondary picture for you, however, you soon snap out of it and return to one of your primary pictures.

Or let us say that you are a couples therapist with a family systems orientation, which, as I see it, means that your primary pictures consist of one or more of the following:

> The "family-homeostasis, identified-patient" picture.
>
> The "pathological-boundaries-and-coalitions (enmeshment-and-disengagement, triangles, differentiation-and-undifferentiation)" picture.
>
> The "paradoxical-interventions (reframing, positive-connotation, prescribing-the-symptom, predicting-a-relapse)" picture.
>
> The "transmission-through-three-generations (making-a-genogram, conducting-family-of-origin-meetings)" picture.
>
> The "deconstructing-and-reconstructing-the-partners'-'stories'-or-views-of-reality" picture.

There you are, adopting some combination of these five pictures, when suddenly you become aware of the disruptive effects of the partners' "you statements." Whatever else the problem may be, you tell yourself—whether a three-generational problem, the result of family homeostasis, or whatever—this couple needs to learn the difference between "I statements" and "you statements." That is not the main thing you do in therapy, but you are not *against* doing it and think it may be useful. For a moment you turn into a behavior therapist and engage in a little communication skills training.

Or let us say that you are a psychodynamically oriented couples therapist, which, as I see it, means that your primary pictures consist of one or a combination of the following:

The "character-defects, developmental-deficits" picture.
The "holdover-from-childhood" picture.
The "people-hold-onto-symptoms-because-they-serve-unconscious-purposes" picture.

There you are, attributing a client's sexual impotence to "character defects" (fear of intimacy), "holdovers from childhood" (unresolved anger at his mother), and "unconscious purposes" (his wish to frustrate, punish, or control his wife). Suddenly he tells you that the problem began when, following an episode of impotence, he worried about its happening again. Immediately you snap into the "Masters-and-Johnson, performance-anxiety, sensate-focus, sex-therapy" picture—a behavior therapy picture. For a moment you become educational and tell the client about performance anxiety. Of course, if you are the kind of psychodynamic therapist who worries about being nonanalytic, or about diluting the transference, you do *not* do this. (If you are enough of that kind of therapist, you probably don't do couples therapy in the first place.)

And now it is possible to understand what happens when, as I have described at the beginning of the chapter, I shift in and out of theories—that is, how I see in turn each of the following as being at the heart of everyone's problems:

Post-traumatic stress disorder.
Unfinished business with parents.
Shame.
Skills deficits.
Addictions.
Conditioned fear.
Biochemical imbalances.

For me, these theories are *secondary* pictures (except for "shame," which, as I describe shortly, is a version of one of my primary pictures). I snap into them when there is immediate suggestive evidence—and I quickly snap out of them. I am particularly likely to snap into secondary pictures when, for the moment, I lack the information, idea, or angle needed to apply my primary pictures.

Some therapists have been searching for ways to integrate the various therapeutic approaches. It is through secondary pictures that an integrating (or at least an intermixing) of them becomes possible. Although a therapist's major commitment may be, for example, to the psychodynamic approach, he or she may temporarily adopt elements from the family systems, cognitive-behavioral, or any other approach—as secondary pictures.

Rejected Pictures

Such integration is limited, however, in part because there is a third type of picture: "rejected pictures."

> *Rejected pictures* are those you do not snap into even if there *is* immediate suggestive evidence for them. Your therapeutic approach is defined, in part, by your rejected pictures—by the pictures you go out of your way *not* to have, and if you find yourself having, you try to shift out of.

The "family-homeostasis, identified-patient" picture is based in part on *not* accepting the "character-defects" picture—that is, on rejecting the family's attribution of the problem to the personal pathology (the character defects) of the identified patient.

The cognitive-behavioral approach is also based in part on not accepting the "character-defects" picture, but in this case the emphasis is on seeing the problem as the result of faulty learning: as skills deficits, as partners' use of aversive rather than positive measures for controlling each other's behavior, and as the result of irrational ideas.

The "Oedipal-wishes" picture is based in part on *not* accepting the "unempathic-or-abusive-parenting" picture—that is, on not accepting the client's view that he or she is a passive victim, but demonstrating to this person that the problem is his or her own Oedipal strivings.

We reject certain primary pictures adopted by therapists from other orientations because they contradict our primary pictures. The therapist with a "family-homeostasis, identified-patient" primary picture views the "character-defects" picture (i.e., accepting the family's attribution of the problem to the pathology or character defects of the identified patient) as colluding with the family to reinforce the pathological family system. Such a therapist sees adopting the "character-defects" picture as countertherapeutic.

Distinguishing among the Three Types of Pictures

All therapists have primary, secondary, and rejected pictures. A quick way to remember these three is that:

> Primary pictures are those you have even without immediate suggestive evidence.
>
> Secondary pictures are those you have only with immediate suggestive evidence.
>
> Rejected pictures are those you reject despite immediate suggestive evidence, because they directly contradict one of more of your primary pictures.

At times—and without knowing it—we snap into secondary pictures that are not congruent with our primary pictures. A psychodynamically oriented therapist, who believes that a husband's premature ejaculation serves the unconscious purpose of wanting to soil his wife or to frustrate her, may nonetheless—and perhaps without recognizing the incongruity—suggest that these partners use the behavior-therapy-oriented squeeze technique. If it is true, as this therapist believes, that the husband's problem is an unconscious wish to soil his wife, it is hard to see how the squeeze technique will help, since it does not deal with this unconscious wish.

At other times—and without knowing it—we snap into one of our *rejected* pictures. Some therapists have the "serves-an-unconscious-purpose, whatever-happens-is-what-the-person-unconsciously-wanted-to-happen" picture as one of their primary pictures; that is, they view people as creating their own destinies and think it naive to see people as victims. The "victim" picture—which, as I describe shortly, is one of my primary pictures—is one of *their* rejected pictures; they see it as countertherapeutic. They are concerned that it may establish a "victim mentality" or reinforce the client's refusal to accept responsibility for his or her behavior. In their clinical work, however—that is, when they have actual people in front of them (particularly certain clients, such as adult children of alcoholics)—these therapists may often appreciate that people are victims. At such moments, they snap into the "victim" picture, but without realizing that they have shifted into one of their rejected pictures and are violating one of their primary pictures.

Reading a book on therapy means reading about the author's particular set of primary, secondary, and rejected pictures. In the next chapter, I describe mine.

CHAPTER 27

The Four Ego-Analytic Pictures

As I have said, every therapist's approach can be described as a combination of primary, secondary, and rejected pictures. Here are my four primary pictures:

1. The "people-generate-symptoms-when-unable-to-get-something-across" picture—which I have dealt with most directly in Chapters 21 through 25.
2. The "hidden-validity" or "focusing-on-what-is-valid-rather-than-on-what-is-invalid-in-the-clients'-responses" picture—which underlies the book as a whole.
3. The "victim-and-joint-victims" picture—which also underlies the book as a whole.
4. The "platform-and-joint-platform" picture—which I have dealt with most directly in Chapters 6 through 8.

Picture 1: The "People-Generate-Symptoms-When-Unable-to-Get-Something-Across" Picture

Even before clients (partners) walk into my office, I am all set to see their problems as a result of an inability to get across leading-edge feelings. I look for what it is—because they are unable to get it across—that has led to the generating of symptoms.

Neil Jacobson, who employs a cognitive-behavioral version of some of the ideas in this book, uses this picture as one of his *secondary* pictures. As a cognitive-behaviorist, he is concerned with teaching needed skills, drawing attention to faulty thinking, and facilitating the partners' use of positive rather than aversive measures for controlling each other's behavior. If a wife comes to a therapy session too upset about an incident that week between herself and her husband to get down to business, Jacobson, in a procedure he calls "troubleshooting" (Jacobson & Holtzworth-Munroe, 1986), interviews her about the incident. Jacobson hopes to give her a chance to have her say—to get across what she needs to—so they can return to the task at hand. For me, helping partners get across what they need to *is* the task at hand. It is one of the *main* things I am doing—it is one of my primary pictures—whereas Jacobson appeals to it when the main thing he is doing is not working.[1]

I have used the expression "becoming symptomatic" to describe the result of failing to get across leading-edge feelings. But what does "becoming symptomatic" really mean? It means "having a tantrum." When people are unable to get across their leading-edge feeling, it is eventually going to burst through. That is what a tantrum is—an eruption of suppressed feeling. The eruption may take the form of an explosion, or it may be a sputter or a whine. As I see it, all of us are always on the verge of a tantrum, although we don't know we are and, to the extent that we do, we think we shouldn't be.

The word "tantrum" has a negative connotation. When people hear it, they think of spoiled children stamping their feet or flying into rages. I use the word, despite its negative connotation, because it so instantly brings to mind—better than any other word I know—a bursting through of suppressed feeling. I want to suggest that tantrums can happen at any moment, about anything, and to anyone—adult or child. In the standard type of tantrum, commonly called "throwing a fit," the person flies into a rage, calls names, yells, lashes out, or even hurls objects across the room. But there are other kinds of tantrums:

The 1-second tantrum—blurting something out.

The subdued or covert tantrum—saying something under your breath, making a face, wrinkling your brow.

The sophisticated tantrum—a sarcastic remark, an elegant putdown.

The silent tantrum—sulking, withdrawing, finding yourself with nothing to say.

The "drawing-the-wagons-into-a-circle" tantrum—becoming defensive, narrowed-down, and grim.

The "becoming-anxious-and-panicky" tantrum.

The "chicken-with-its-head-cut-off" tantrum—becoming flustered, confused, or disorganized; desperately trying to fix the situation.

---

[1] Christensen, Jacobson, and Babcock (in press) will shortly publish an updated behavioral couples therapy approach that has even closer correspondences to many of the ideas in this book.

The "exaggerated-compliance/exaggerated-solution" tantrum—"Well, if you don't like my friends, I'll never invite anyone over ever again"; "If you object to my watching *Monday Night Football*, maybe we should get a divorce."

How does having the "people-generate-symptoms/throw-a-tantrum-when-unable-to-get-something-across" primary picture affect my therapeutic work? To a large extent, it *is* my therapeutic work. At any given moment when doing therapy, I am looking to see what my client—and, in couples therapy, what each partner—needs to get across to become tantrum-free (i.e., symptom-free).

Picture 2: The "Focusing-on-What-Is-Valid-Rather-Than-on-What-Is-Invalid-in-the-Clients'-Responses" Picture

The full title of this second picture is the "feeling-of-unentitlement, making-clients'-cases-for-them, noticing-what-is-valid-rather-than-what-is-invalid-in-their-responses" picture. For simplicity I refer to it as the "noticing-what-is-valid-in-the-clients'-responses" or simply the "hidden-validity" picture. This picture is a crucial one, so I devote a large part of the chapter to it.

Here is the idea behind this important picture. As a result of believing they are unentitled to their feelings, people are unable to make their own best case—that is, to talk about their experience in a way that would get others to sympathize with them and to appreciate how they feel. When they manage to reach out to others and try to make their case anyway, they do so in inhibited, indirect, awkward, desperate, pressured, offensive, explosive, and counterproductive ways—for example, by whining, demanding, and withdrawing.

The therapist's job is:

1. To recognize that clients' offensive behavior is a consequence of their feeling unentitled to their feelings and their resulting inability to make their case.
2. To help clients make their case and—by demonstrating how much better a position it puts them in—to let them see that the problem to a large extent is their *inability* to make their case.
3. To show what it would look like if clients *were* to feel entitled to their feelings and—by demonstrating how much better a position it puts them in (i.e., how it allows productive thinking, talking, and problem solving)—to reveal that the problem to a large extent is their feeling *un*entitled to their feelings.

As I hope is clear, my goal is not necessarily to *increase* clients' sense of entitlement to feelings—although, of course, I would be pleased if this were to happen. Feeling entitled to feelings is difficult and to some extent impossible. We keep stumbling into feelings that we are ashamed of; that is, that we judge ourselves to be weak, bad, irrational, crazy, immature, unmanly, or unfeminine for having. Such judgments represent ways of feeling unentitled.

More possible, although still difficult, is to create a platform from which to monitor our shifting sense of entitlement to our feelings. As I have discussed earlier, creating such a platform in therapy—that is, enabling clients to sympathize with themselves for feeling unentitled to their feelings—is itself a type of solution.

To do the three things I have described above—to show that the problem is our clients' inability to make their case, to help them make it, and to show what it would look like if they felt entitled to their feelings—requires that the therapist counteract the clients' tendencies to invalidate their case. It requires that the therapist focus on what is valid in clients' responses. And that is why I call it the "feeling-of-unentitlement, making-clients'-cases-for-them, noticing-what-is-valid-rather-than-what-is-invalid-in-the-clients' responses" picture.

As I see it, and as I have described it most directly in Chapters 4 and 5, everyone's big problem is feeling unentitled to feelings. I have talked about it throughout the book, referring to it variously as "self-accusation," "self-blame," "negative self-talk," the "harsh internal taskmaster," the "non-self-sympathetic" state of mind, "self-doubt," "self-suspicion," "self-prejudice," "self-condemnation," and "self-hate." And I could also have used the words "guilt," "shame," "punitive superego," "narcissistic vulnerability," "sense of unworthiness," and "sense of sin."

Even before clients walk into my office, I am all set to see their problems as the consequences of feeling unentitled to their feelings. In practice, this means being prepared to notice the effects on them of the following:

Their self-reproach.

Their battle with their harsh internal taskmasters.

Their struggle for self-justification: They fight off their taskmasters' moral injunctions with moral injunctions of their own.

Their blame of others (in an effort to get the blame off themselves).

Their inability to know what they feel: Their concern about what they should and shouldn't feel makes it hard for them to know what they do feel.

Their inability to think: Their concern what they should and shouldn't do, think, and feel makes it hard for them to think in a neutral, unbiased, nonjudgmental, objective, "just-trying-to-find-the-facts, just-looking-for-the-truth, not-having-to-prove-anything, not-having-to-do-anything-about-it" manner.

As a result of their self-reproach—and impeded by their long list of shoulds and shouldn'ts—clients often behave in inhibited, indirect, offensive, provocative, and unattractive ways that alienate others and lead others to side against them.

In a word, clients are typically unable to make their case, to state their point of view convincingly, to represent their position in ways that get others to appreciate how they feel. In their abortive efforts to make their case, they behave in bullying, nagging, whining, angry, or morally judgmental ways that turn others against them.

My job in therapy (individual, couples, or any other kind) is to help clients make their case: to represent their positions in a better way than they are able to do themselves. My job in couples therapy is to help both partners make their case—to develop both partners' positions simultaneously. The task, as Apfelbaum (1982b) wrote, is to serve as a lawyer hired by both partners.

In my effort to make my clients' case, I find that certain classic psychotherapeutic ideas (or, as I call them here, "pictures")—ideas that many of us subscribe to and find useful—can at times be more of a hindrance than a help. These include the "character-defects, developmental-deficits," "holdover-from-childhood," "serves-a-hidden-purpose," "bad-habits," and "irrational-ideas" pictures.

Let us say that in a couples therapy session, Marie and Paul describe the following event from the previous evening. Marie, who is usually on time—and, in general, is a considerate and conscientious person—phoned Paul to say that she was going to be a little late getting home. Paul exploded:

> Why bother to come home at all? I've never seen anyone so irresponsible. Do you ever think of anybody but yourself? No wonder I can't count on you for anything. When are you going to notice that there's someone else in this relationship? You never think about me at all.

One common psychotherapeutic picture—Bacon's primary picture—is the "character-defects, developmental-deficits" picture. In adopting this picture, the therapist looks to see how the client's symptomatic behavior is a consequence of his or her immaturity, developmental deficits, ego defects, regressive impulses, primitive defenses, reduced level of functioning, pathology, and so on. Since Paul's outburst was irrational and overblown—and since, let us say, it was just the latest in a series of such tantrum-like explosions—such a therapist takes it as further evidence that Paul has a personality disorder, with possible borderline or narcissistic traits (he gets upset if he does not get his way).

But there is a problem. Once you adopt the "character-defects, developmental-deficits" picture and attribute Paul's outburst to his borderline or narcissistic tendencies, you will have discredited his behavior—and to some extent Paul himself—and you will see it as of secondary importance that he might have had reason for being angry at Marie. You will consider it a technical error to become too caught up in the precipitating event and to fail to place your emphasis where it belongs: on the character defect. For someone like me, who sees the problem as clients' feeling unentitled to their feelings—and, in particular, as the ways that people *already* reproach themselves (and one another) for their character defects—it is a technical error to fail to check out the possibility that this "character defect" (Paul's eruptive and overblown response; i.e., his tantrum-like explosion) might be a result of feeling unentitled to a feeling.

> To a therapist who focuses on character defects, Paul's eruptive and overblown response would be a direct expression of a character defect.
>
> To a therapist like me, Paul's eruptive and overblown response would be a reaction to an inhibition—a consequence of feeling unentitled to an ordinary feeling.

What was the "ordinary feeling" to which Paul felt unentitled in this instance? One possibility might be his wish that Marie comfort him about his bad day. Since he felt unentitled to this wish, he would have been unable to tell her about this wish or even to remain aware of it himself. He would have been left with a vague sense of wanting something from Marie, but not knowing what, and feeling frustrated for not getting it. Marie's telling him she was going to be late might have provided the peg on which Paul hung this frustration, and perhaps he blew up at her as a result.

Another common psychotherapeutic picture—Farland's primary picture—is the "holdover-from-childhood" picture. Here the therapist looks for ways in which the present is a metaphor for the past. If you are this kind of therapist, and you hear that Paul's father left for military service when Paul was only 5, you consider the possibility that Paul's anger at Marie was a displacement of anger at his father for abandoning him. Perhaps Marie's lateness simply reminded Paul of this abandonment. If you suggest to Paul that his grudge might be more with his father than with Marie, you may defuse the situation. And this clearly will be useful—at least to the extent that Paul's anger at Marie *was* affected by his unresolved feelings toward his father.

But there is a danger. Once you adopt the "holdover-from-childhood" picture and place your emphasis on how Paul's anger at Marie was a displacement of anger toward his father long ago:

> You may easily lose interest in looking for how Paul might have had reason for being angry at her last night.
>
> And you may easily lose interest in asking questions (e.g., "Paul, how were you feeling just *before* Marie's called to say she was going to be late?") that could reveal how his behavior might have been a response to what was happening at the moment.

A third common psychotherapeutic picture—Eberheart's primary picture—is the "serves-a-function, the-person-must-have-wanted-it-that-way, holding-onto-symptoms-because-they-serve-unconscious-purposes" picture. In adopting it, the therapist looks for what the client may be getting from the symptom, and, in particular, how this symptomatic behavior may allow the client to manipulate others, control relationships, and gratify regressive needs. If you are this kind of therapist and observe that Paul's irrational anger led to a fight, you consider the possibility that Paul might have *wanted* the fight in order to protect himself against too much intimacy.

But, again, there is a problem. Once you adopt the "serves-a-purpose, the-person-must-have-wanted-it-that-way" picture and see Paul as getting what he wanted and as unconsciously controlling what went on, it becomes hard to see that he might not at all be getting what he wants from this and similar incidents—that he hates the fight even though it was his own actions that started it; that he is a victim of the fight he started. If you are operating from a "serves-a-purpose" picture, you think it naive to see people as victims.

A fourth common psychotherapeutic picture—Greenholtz's primary picture—is the "bad-habits, skills-deficits" picture. Here the therapist looks for how the symptom results from skills deficits, information deficits, conditioned fear, maladaptive reinforcement contingencies, nonoptimal forms of learning (such as partners' use of aversive rather than positive means to control each other's behavior), and so on. If you are this kind of therapist, since Marie and Paul were unable to talk things out and instead got into a fight, you conclude that they need communication training. And since Paul exploded when Marie told him she was going to be late, you conclude that he was trying to control her behavior—to get her to think twice before coming home late again by punishing her for being late this time.

The problem is this: Once you adopt the "bad-habits, skills-deficits, nonoptimal-ways-of-controlling-other-people's-behavior" picture and see Paul as violating the rules of good communication, blaming rather than being reasonable, and using punishment rather than positive reinforcement to control Marie's behavior, it becomes difficult to see how it might have made *sense* for him to violate the rules of good communication and to punish rather than use positive reinforcement. Once you have a picture of how you think partners *should* behave:

> You may easily lose interest in exploring how the ways they *do* behave make sense.
>
> You may easily believe that you should promote this behavior and that people should be able to adopt it.

The fifth common psychotherapeutic picture—Albert Ellis's primary picture—is the "irrational-ideas, unrealistic-expectations, cognitive-restructuring" picture. In adopting this picture, the therapist looks for faulty ideas, irrational beliefs, negative self-talk, faulty assumptions, pathogenic beliefs, fantasy-based expectations, stories, or covert couple rules or myths that might underlie and cause the symptom. The therapist then disputes these irrational ideas. In this case, Paul appears to have the irrational idea that Marie should devote herself entirely to his wishes. The therapeutic task, accordingly, is to get Paul to see that *he* is responsible for his own happiness and that it is unrealistic of him to depend on Marie for it.

But once you adopt the "unrealistic-expectations" picture and see Paul as expecting Marie to devote himself entirely to his needs, it becomes difficult to see that he might be expecting her to satisfy hardly *any* of them. He might be making a stand on trivial issues such as Marie's being a little late because he is unable to make a stand on really *important* issues, such as feeling taken for granted or feeling a lack of intimacy in the relationship.

The problem with these five common psychotherapeutic ideas (pictures) is that:

> They so convincingly demonstrate how clients' responses are *in*valid that it becomes hard to think of how they *might* be valid.
>
> They so effectively direct our thinking to how the clients' reactions do not make sense in the present situation that we can easily overlook how they *might* make sense.

I want to look at how these responses might make sense in the present situation because, according to my primary picture—the "noticing-what-is-valid-in-the-clients'-responses" primary picture—problems arise from clients' *own* feelings that their responses are invalid and do not make sense; that is, they arise from their feeling of unentitlement to or self-reproach about their responses. The problem with such self-reproach, as I have said, is that it blocks constructive thinking, talking, and problem solving.

These five common psychotherapeutic pictures—to the extent that they cause me to focus my attention on what is invalid in clients' responses and thus lead me to violate my "focus-on-what's-valid-in-clients'-responses" primary picture—are among my rejected pictures. Whenever I find that my use of one of these five pictures causes me to focus too much on what is invalid in clients' responses, I try to compensate by looking for:

1. A hidden appropriateness.
2. A provocation that the client's childhood-based special sensitivity enables him or her to detect.
3. An underlying ordinary feeling.
4. Important information about the relationship for which the irrational-appearing behavior is a useful rough first approximation—that is, a clue.
5. A universal issue.

I go over these rules of thumb one at a time.

• **Rule of Thumb 1: A hidden appropriateness.** I look for a hidden appropriateness in the client's seemingly inappropriate response.

Paul's outburst seemed *in*appropriate because it was apparently *un*provoked—it seemed to come out of nowhere. So I look for a hidden way in which it *might* have been provoked.

When Marie told Paul that she was going to be a little late, she said it nervously, as if he were a difficult person who had to be handled carefully. So that is what upset him—not her being late, but the nervous way she told him about it. *Anyone* might be upset by that.

• **Rule of Thumb 2: A provocation that the person's childhood-based special sensitivity enables him or her to detect.** I try to see how the client may be reacting—although with a historically based special sensitivity—to an immediate provocation.

In using Rule of Thumb 2 in this case, I start out by accepting the view that Paul has a special sensitivity to abandonment based on his father's going overseas. But—and it is an important *but*—I then assume that Paul's sensitivity to abandonment was being activated in direct response to something happening at the moment. Marie *was* abandoning him. Her treating him as someone she could not confide in and had to "handle" *was* an abandonment—albeit a subtle one.

• **Rule of Thumb 3: An underlying ordinary feeling.** I look for an ordinary feeling that the client is expressing in an indirect and offensive way (e.g., suppressing it and then blurting it out) because he or she feels unentitled to it.

Paul has been feeling a little taken for granted recently—that is the ordinary feeling. He was previously unable to tell Marie about it, however, because he felt his feeling was unjustified. He had nothing concrete to point to. Marie's calling to say she was going to be a little late—as minor an infraction as this might seem—provided him with something concrete to point to, and all his pent-up anger about feeling taken for granted came bursting forth.

• **Rule of Thumb 4: Important information about the relationship for which the irrational-appearing behavior is a useful rough first approximation.** I look to see how the client's exaggerated or symptomatic reaction may be a response to—and a potential clue to—an important feeling or issue in the relationship.

Marie and Paul might wish that he did *not* have a sensitivity to abandonment. It is a nuisance that he gets upset at even minor slights. His sensitivity has at least one important benefit, however. Marie and Paul will never wake up one day, as some people do, and find themselves in a detached, withdrawn relationship without knowing how they got there. Paul is their protection against that. He is an expert at detecting the subtle and often unnoticed slights and rejections that regularly occur between people.

• **Rule of Thumb 5: A universal issue.** I look to see whether the client may simply be experiencing a clear and intensified form of a common (universal) problem—that is, a problem with which to one degree or another nearly everyone (and every couple) struggles.

Paul might be experiencing an intense version of the common couple problem of accountability—that is, the degree to which partners are free to do what they want versus the degree to which they should take into account each other's wishes.

With the aid of these five rules of thumb, I am able to focus on what is valid rather than what is invalid in the clients' responses. This helps in at least two major ways:

First, I now have something to tell clients. If I operate from, say, a "character-defects, developmental-deficits" picture with Paul and see him as suffering from a narcissistic or borderline personality disorder, it is hard to think of what I could tell him that he wouldn't experience as a putdown—that is, that would not just threaten or demoralize him and increase his resistance. But if I notice what is valid rather than what is invalid in his responses—if I see his position as making even more sense than *he* does—then I have plenty to tell him.

How do therapists with a "character-defects, developmental-defects" primary picture deal with the "threatening-and-demoralizing-to-the-clients" nature of their stance? One way (some of them tell me) is to adopt the "focusing-on-what-is-valid-in-the-clients'-responses" picture as a secondary picture. These therapists conceptualize their clients' problems in "character-defects, developmental-deficits" terms. When it comes to actually saying something to their clients, however, they shift temporarily into the "focusing-on-what-is-valid-in-the-clients'-responses" picture.

The second major way in which focusing on what is valid in clients' responses aids in my therapeutic work is by protecting me from seeing one partner as right and the other as wrong—a difficult place from which to operate when doing couples therapy. In adopting the "noticing-what-is-valid-in-the-clients'-responses" primary picture, I assume that each partner's position makes sense, even if at first it may not seem to. In fact, that is the major thing I am doing as a couples therapist: developing each partner's position to show how it makes sense.

I have said that the five common psychotherapeutic pictures are to some extent my rejected pictures. I don't mean to dismiss them entirely, however. People *do*, after all, have character defects; their problems do go back to childhood; they do obtain secondary gain from their symptoms; and they do have skills deficits, bad habits, and unrealistic expectations. So I need a way to incorporate the five common psychotherapeutic ideas into my thinking—but in a manner that doesn't conflict with my primary pictures.

The problem is not the five common psychotherapeutic pictures in themselves, but how they are used. They run the risk—in addition to preventing me from seeing how my clients' behavior *may* make sense—of being employed in the service of the clients' self-hate and blocking me from seeing clients as people with whom I can collaborate.

My ways to reduce this risk are:

To use these five common psychotherapeutic ideas as *secondary* pictures rather than as primary pictures.
To use them, as much as possible, in the *service* of my primary pictures.
To make sure that they do not slide over into becoming what for me are *rejected* pictures—that is, to make sure that my use of them does not violate my primary pictures.

For example, when Paul's associations in the therapy session go back to his feelings about his father's being called up for military duty, I join him in the "holdover-from-childhood" picture. For several minutes we look at how his anger at Marie's being a little late was connected with his anger at his father long ago. Paul is relieved by the idea that his anger might really be at his father. He doesn't like feeling angry at Marie; it makes him feel too alienated from her. I am using what is for me a secondary picture—the "holdover-from-childhood" picture—in the service of creating a joint platform: a "sympathizing-with-one-another" vantage point from which Paul and Marie can appreciate what *he* had to deal with in childhood and what *she* has to deal with because of his childhood.

But suddenly Paul gets a sour look on his face. And when I ask him about it, he says that he feels we are blaming everything on him; by tracing his anger to feelings about his father, we are saying that his anger at Marie is unjustified.

This means that Paul believes that *I* believe that the crucial point is his distortion of the present in terms of the past. Paul doesn't realize (because I haven't gotten to it yet) that the crucial point for me is how his childhood-based special sensitivities enable him to detect a present provocation.

My "holdover-from-childhood" reasoning, which a moment ago was serving the purposes of my "create-a-platform" primary picture, is, *in Paul's eyes*, now causing me to focus on what is invalid in his reactions, placing me in violation of my "focus-on-what-is-valid-in-clients'-reactions" primary picture. For a moment, "holdover-from-childhood" is functioning as a rejected picture.

So, to refocus on what is *valid* in Paul's reactions, I suggest that the obvious and traumatic way in which Paul was abandoned by his father in the past may provide him with a clearer version of how he felt more subtly abandoned by Marie last night. And he *was* being abandoned by Marie last night. As I have said above, the cautious way in which she felt it necessary to tell him that she was going to be late—as if he were a difficult person whose feelings she had to manage—*was* an abandonment, although of a less dramatic kind.

In so saying, I shift:

From *the "Holdover-from-Childhood" Picture, in Which:*	To *the "Noticing-What-Is-Valid-in-Paul's-Responses" Picture, in Which:*
1. The past is used to invalidate the present: Paul's reactions are seen as hangups from childhood.	1. The past is used to reveal a truth about the present—that is, to disclose and dramatize what is happening in the present.
2. The present is seen as a metaphor for the past.	2. The past is seen as a metaphor for the present.
3. The present is viewed as a good way to see what happened in the past. The focus is on reconstructin the past.	3. The past is viewed as a good way to see what is happening in the present. The focus is on explicating the present.

To summarize my relationship with the five common psychotherapeutic pictures (i.e., the "character-defects," "holdover-from-childhood," "serves-a-purpose," "bad-habits," and "irrational-ideas" pictures):

> These five are to some extent among my rejected pictures, since, by focusing on what is invalid in the clients' responses, they contradict one of my primary pictures: the "noticing-what-is-valid-in-my-clients'-responses" primary picture.
> Because I find myself at times adopting them, I need the rules of thumb to extricate myself.
> But since there is something about each of these five common psychotherapeutic pictures that is clearly useful, I include them also among my secondary pictures.
> In fact, at times certain of these five operate in the *service* of my primary pictures.

Picture 3: The "Victim-and-Joint-Victims" Primary Picture

Even before clients walk into my office, I am all set to see them as "victims"—and, in the case of partners, as "joint victims." I know this puts me out of step with the modern (and also classic) emphasis on self-responsibility, so I had better explain myself.

First, let me acknowledge that the self-responsibility ethic can be liberating and empowering:

You are in a better position to deal with relationship problems if you focus on how you can change rather than on how your *part-ner* can change (since you typically have only limited power to get your partner to change). For example, you are likely to engage in less spinning of your wheels if you realize that your efforts to help your alcoholic spouse are likely to be counterproductive; that is, you can only take responsibility for yourself, and your alcoholic spouse can only take responsibility for himself or herself.

You may feel less powerless in the face of a disease such as cancer if you feel that you are not a helpless victim, but can control the course of the disease by, for example, imagery, will power, the way you eat, or the way you live.

But the self-responsibility ethic can also be demoralizing and *disem*powering:

When (as at times you inevitably will do) you snap into a "feeling-I-can't-do-it-by-myself, needing-my-partner-to-change" state of mind, you will feel that you are doing something wrong; that you are having the wrong wishes, feelings, and needs; that you are violating the self-responsibility ethic. And you will feel bad about it. And, feeling bad, you will be blocked from productive thinking, collaborating, and problem solving.

When (as at times you inevitably will do) you will try to help your alcoholic spouse (it is sometimes unbearable to stand by and see someone you care about self-destruct without trying to do something about it), you will feel that you are doing something wrong— that you are a coalcoholic, a codependent, and an enabler. And your energies will be sidetracked into feeling bad about it.

When you feel responsible for your cancer, you have to deal not only with the disease itself but with the belief that it is your own fault for getting it, or at least for not overcoming it.

The major problem with the self-responsibility ethic is this demoralizing and disempowering effect. It can easily foster the kind of "self-accusing, suspicious-of-myself, it's-my-own-responsibility, I've-got-to-be-careful-not-to-let-myself-off-too-easy, it's-my-own-fault, I-have-only-myself-to-blame" attitude that we have too much of already and that I see as the root of our problems.

As I have said, everyone's big problem is self-reproach—and, more generally, feeling unentitled to his or her feelings—which interferes with the ability to think, talk, and solve problems. The self-responsibility ethic, since it *is* an ethic (i.e., a set of moral precepts establishing how a person should and shouldn't behave, think, or feel), enforces and embodies certain self-reproachful ideas. The client feels:

It's my own fault; I'm doing it to myself.

I'm sitting here feeling sorry for myself and blaming others rather than making an effort to change.

I could change if I wanted to and the fact that I don't must mean I'm getting something out of it.

The self-responsibility ethic is the second in a one–two punch. "There is something wrong with me" is the first punch. "And I've got no one to blame but myself" is the second.

Eberheart's primary picture—the "serves-a-purpose, the-person-must-have-wanted-it-that-way" picture—is built on the self-responsibility ethic. Whatever happens, Eberheart believes, is what the person (at least unconsciously) wants to happen. There are no accidents. There are no unintended consequences. There are no victims—only perpetrators.

I believe, on the other hand, that:

There are accidents.

There are unintended consequences—Marie and Paul's evening can be thought of as an uninterrupted series of unintended consequences.

There are victims—in the case of couple relationships, there are two victims.

It is easy in couples therapy, particularly when one partner is less skillful than the other in presenting his or her position, to see that partner as the perpetrator and the other as the victim. It is difficult at such a moment to remember that everyone is a victim.

To remind myself, I adopt the "victim" picture—in couples therapy, the "joint-victims" picture—as one of my primary pictures. The "victim-and-joint-victims" primary picture predisposes me to see how clients can be in trapped, stuck, "back-against-the-wall" positions, even if it does not look that way.

In adopting the "victim-and-joint-victims" picture, I focus on how clients are stuck (deprived, cornered, getting little or nothing from their symptoms) rather than on how they are gratified (getting secondary gain, unconsciously designing their destinies and controlling the situation, getting too much from their symptoms to want to give them up)—which is how I would see them were I operating from Eberheart's "serves-a-purpose" picture.

Eberheart's view is thus for me a rejected picture. In fact, it is my major rejected picture—which is probably apparent from what I have already said. If Eberheart were to write this book, she would not have based it, as I have done, on a fine-grained analysis of Marie and Paul's half-thoughts and half-feelings. Eberheart would see such an analysis as unnecessary; she would feel she has already drawn all the information she needs from the behavioral outcome. If you believe with Eberheart that whatever happens is what the person at least unconsciously wants to happen, then all you need to do is notice what happens and draw the obvious conclusions:

> Since Marie's immediately telling Paul about her bad day alienated him, Eberheart would conclude that Marie must have *wanted* to alienate him—perhaps so that she could justify feeling misunderstood by him, or so that she could protect herself against too much intimacy.
>
> Since Paul's escaping to watch the News provoked a fight, Eberheart would conclude that Paul must have *wanted* to provoke a fight—perhaps so that he could take out on Marie his frustrations from the day, or so that *he* could protect himself against too much intimacy.

If, like Eberheart, you have the "serves-a-purpose, the-person-must-have-wanted-it-that-way" picture, all you need to do is notice what ultimately happens and infer intention from effect.

Many therapists hesitate to think of clients as victims. (For example, clients who as children were sexually abused by a parent are described as "incest survivors" rather than as "incest victims.") They are concerned that their clients not develop a "victim mentality," by which they mean a "feeling-hopeless, helpless, resigned, self-blaming, it's ultimately-my-own-fault, I-deserve-what-I-get" state of mind. Here is my response to that. By enabling clients to see themselves as victims:

> I mean helping them develop an ability to sympathize with themselves (rather than to blame themselves) for what they are stuck in.
>
> I specifically do *not* mean developing a "victim mentality," since it prominently features self-blame (i.e., "it's ultimately my own fault, I deserve what I get").

A "victim mentality" is itself something that people may easily get stuck in. So whan I say I try to enble people to see themselves as victims—by which I mean help them sympathize with themselves for what they are stuck in—I include helping them sympathize with themselves for being stuck in (i.e., for having difficulty freeing themselves from) a "victim mentality."

In fact, rescuing people from the self-blame generated by seeing themselves as having a "victim mentality" is a major purpose of the "victim" picture. Here again clients are subject to a one-two punch. The first punch is having to suffer the effects of being a victim. The second punch is reproaching themselves for having a "victim mentality"—that is, for any tendency they have to feel helpless, hopeless, resigned, and so on.

The purpose of the "victim" picture is thus threefold. It is to help the therapist realize (or remember) that clients suffer from:

1. The self-responsibility ethic—their tendency to blame them-selves for their problems ("It's my own fault; I'm doing it to my-self").
2. Failure to realize or appreciate that they are victims—that they are deprived, stuck, and trapped.
3. Self-blame for having a "victim mentality."

Why have I chosen the graphic and shocking word "victim" to define this primary picture, rather than some word that is less provoca-tive, less controversial, and less burdened with unwanted connotations, such as "stuck," "trapped," or "deprived"?

To distinguish it more clearly from—and to show how incompat-ible it is with—the "serves-a-purpose, the-person-must-have-wanted-it-that-way" picture and with the self-responsibility ethic.

To emphasize that part of the problem is the client's self-criticism that he or she has a victim mentality.

When I say that partners are joint victims, do I mean that a physi-cally abusing husband is a victim? Yes. As is well known, many physi-cally abusing partners were themselves physically abused as children. As is also well known, the typical abusing or battering husband is an extreme example of a person who is aggressive because he cannot be assertive; that is, he has difficulty holding up his end in an argument. He strikes out physically when he feels helpless in the face of his wife's verbal attack, real or imagined.

Even though I see the battering husband as a victim himself, I must state two important qualifications. The first is that until the abuse has stopped, there is no way to *care* whether the husband himself is a vic-tim. Our first priority has to be the wife's safety and her feelings—how she feels terrorized, how she blames herself, how the abuse undermines her self-esteem. Unless the therapist attends to these feelings, a battered woman may be unable to extricate herself from an abusive situation; attending to her feelings may free her to free herself.

The second qualification arises from the confusion between "understanding" and "excusing." Or, to put it another way, at issue here are two meanings of the word "understanding." The wife's and the therapist's *understanding* the physically abusing husband in the sense of recognizing that he himself is a victim does not mean that she and the therapist have to be *understanding* in the sense of excusing, forgiving, accepting, or putting up with the abuse.

Too often, the victim of battering does confuse understanding with excusing. She confuses the two when she tells herself, "Poor guy, he can't help himself, so I don't have the right to leave him." She thinks she has to excuse him, forgive him, or tolerate his behavior. She would *not* be confusing understanding with excusing were she to say to herself, "Poor guy, he can't help himself, but I don't care; I hate him," or "Poor guy, he can't help himself, but I can help *myself*; I'm leaving."

Picture 4: The "Platform-and-Joint-Platform" Picture

Even before clients walk into my office, I am all set to see their problems as resulting from the lack of a platform from which to manage their lives and their relationships. Without such a platform, they are unable to think anything through, and the situation quickly deteriorates.

As I have emphasized throughout this chapter (and this book), everyone's big problem is self-reproach—or, more generally, feeling unentitled to his or her feelings. In creating a platform, you become a one-person consciousness-raising group (or, with your partner, a two-person group) for dealing with the following:

Feeling unentitled to your feelings.
Your problems.
The prejudices that you have against yourself and that others (or society) have against you.
The occupational hazards of being a human being.
The occupational hazards of being in a relationship.

Your attention is no longer on the problem itself, but the conversation you are having with yourself or with your partner *about* the problem. Membership in this consciousness-raising group *is* the solution to the problem.

Creating a platform is itself the solution to problems—or at least to *some* kinds of problems:

Creating a joint platform is *not* a solution when the problem is, for example, that one partner wants to have children and the other does not.

Creating a joint platform *is* the solution when the problem is the fights the partners get into when they try to talk about whether to have children.

Creating a platform is the solution when the absence of a neutral, nonaccusing vantage point from which to think about and discuss the problem is the problem.

In talks I give to therapists about my approach, I am typically asked, "After you get your client on the platform, what do you do next? How do you really solve the problem?" When I hear that, I know that I have not gotten across what the platform is. The platform is a new, second-order, overarching perspective that in itself may be the solution. The platform is not a means to an end—it *is* the end.

At a certain point in the session described earlier in this chapter, Paul's attention is on the problem, which he defines as his sensitivity to abandonment. Here Paul is adopting the "holdover-from-childhood" definition of the problem. He sees his problem as baggage from childhood that he should take care of on his own.

So I try to give Paul a glimpse of the platform definition of the problem. Here the problem is viewed, not as Paul's childhood-based special sensitivity to abandonment, but as how he relates to himself (and to Marie) about his sensitivity to abandonment.

For Paul, "being on the platform" means the following:

Being able to think (and talk with Marie) about the problem rather than immediately having to solve it, and, failing that, giving up on it entirely and pretending it doesn't exist.

Having an ongoing way to think (and talk with Marie) about the problem and, in the process, to continue developing new information about it.

Taking (or jointly taking) the problem into account—keeping tabs on it, anticipating it, and planning for it—rather than just hoping it will not recur and being unprepared when it does.

So, what *do* I say when therapists ask, "After you get your client on the platform, what do you do next? How do you really solve the problem?" I answer that being on a platform *is* the "next." It's my backup plan. It's what I turn to when I have difficulty applying my original plan, which, like the approach of nearly every other therapist, is to eliminate the problem. *Many* of the problems for which clients seek our help are difficult or impossible to solve. That is where the platform comes in. Creating a platform is the premier way to deal with difficult- or impossible-to-solve problems. By creating a platform, you solve a problem by inhabiting it—that is, by establishing on ongoing, developing, compassionate conversation/relationship with yourself about it.

Sometimes a client says, "I'm on the platform all the time, but my partner never is. I'm tired of its always having to be up to me." Such a person is expressing a weariness, a resentment, and a feeling that he or she is in it all alone—and, of course, that is what I want to focus on. But I doubt that this person is, as he or she says, "on the platform all the time." Being on the platform is a rare event. It is hard to get on it, and it's easy to fall off. We can easily think we are on the platform—that we are being objective, neutral, nonjudgmental, nonaccusing, nondefensive, and so on—when we are not.

The "platform" is my word for what other therapists refer to as, among other things, "neutrality," "objectivity," and "nonjudgmentalness." I use this word because these other more familiar words do not adequately convey the difficulty of the task. We think that all it takes for a therapist to be neutral, objective, and nonjudgmental is to avoid becoming emotionally caught up in the situation (i.e., to avoid countertransference). An advantage of the term "platform" *is* the fact that it is less familiar than these other terms. When you hear it, you hesitate for a moment. And in that moment, I can rush in and show you how complex and difficult an achievement it really is to be neutral, objective, and nonjudgmental.

Actually, the term "platform" does not adequately convey the difficulty of the task either; you think that all you have to do is to "step onto the platform." But at least using the term gives me that momentary pause, so I can rush in with a fuller definition.

And here it is: "Being on the platform" means having the following complex set of awarenesses, understandings, attitudes, and abilities. It is a long list, so I have divided it into several parts. Its very length again dramatizes how difficult an achievement it really is to be "neutral" or "objective." Since a therapist's conception of objectivity depends to some extent on his or her theory, some of the items on this list—items 10–14 in particular—are specific to my theory.

Having a Particular Approach toward Problems

"Being on the platform (or joint platform)" means having a particular approach toward problems. We know we are on the platform if:

1. We think something through, whereas what we typically do is appeal to slogans ("You only think of yourself") and selected facts ("I remember when you . . .") in order to try to prove, justify, or talk ourselves or our partners into or out of something.

2. We think (talk) *about* the problem. What we typically do is unknowingly continue to think (talk) from *within* it.

3. We sit with a problem. What we typically do is feel we have to do something about the problem—solve it, deny that it is a problem, or resign ourselves to it.

4. We experience a sense of relief, power, freedom, enthusiasm, and spirit in being able to focus on (or get through to others about) the problem. What we typically do is experience a sense of struggle, effortfulness, sluggishness, doggedness, and tedium ("Why do we have to do this? Do we always have to talk about every problem?").

Having a Certain Type of Conversation

"Being on the *joint* platform" means having a certain type of conversation. We know we are on a joint platform if we and our partners do the following:

5. We have a developing conversation over time. What we typically do is have the same conversation (or argument) over and over again; fail to talk about the issue at all; or expect to solve the problem in a single discussion and, when we cannot, feel hopeless about it.

6. We talk collaboratively. What we typically do is shift in and out of argument (or continually argue), often without knowing it. If we do know we are arguing (e.g., blaming), we think our partners should not be bothered by it—that they should be able to overlook it.

7. We build on what our partners say. What we typically do is simply agree or disagree.

8. We deal with fights by having recovery conversations. What we typically do is wake up the next morning and try to go on as if nothing has happened.

Having Usable Knowledge of the Four Primary Pictures

"Being on the platform (or joint platform)" means having usable knowledge of all four of my primary pictures. We know we are on the platform if:

9. We recognize that our (or our partners') immature or irrational behavior is a consequence of an inability to get something across—that is, we adopt the "need-to-get-something-across" picture. This contrasts with what we typically believe, which is that we (or they) are simply immature or irrational.

10. We see the validity in both our own and our partners' positions—that is, we adopt the "hidden-validity" primary picture. This contrasts with what we typically do, which is to disqualify our own and/or our partners' positions. We know we are on the platform if we are able to appreciate our partners' point of view without having to give up our own; what we typically do is to blame ourselves or, if not, blame our partners.

11. We see ourselves and our partners as caught in something (as victims)—that is, we adopt the "victim-and-joint-victims" primary picture. This contrasts with what we often do, which is to blame ourselves and/or our partners for our problems.

12. We recognize that the problem is not just the problem in itself, but how we relate to ourselves (and to our partners) about the problem—that is, we adopt the "platform-and-joint-platform" primary picture. This contrasts with what we typically do, which is to believe that the problem *is* just the problem in itself. We know we are on the platform if we realize that much of the problem is our inability to "have" the problem—that is, our inability to think about it without anxiously having to solve it right away.

A Short Discourse on Whether
There Is Such a Thing as Feeling Too Entitled

So those are 12 factors that define being on the platform (being neutral, objective, or nonjudgmental). And here is a 13th. We know we are on the platform if:

13. We realize that we suffer from feeling *un*entitled to our feelings, when what we typically think is that we feel *too* entitled to them.

But what about people who, according to the criteria in the DSM-III-R, have a "narcissistic personality disorder," the characteristics of which include a feeling of entitlement—that is, an "unreasonable expectation of specially favorable treatment, e.g., assumes that he or she does not have to wait in line while others must do so" (American Psychiatric Association, 1987, p. 349)? Do I mean to say that these people also suffer from an underlying feeling of *un*entitlement?

Yes. Let us look at Jim, a man who fits the DSM-III-R description of narcissistic personality disorder, and let us study a specific example of his narcissistic behavior. Jim interrupts a friend, who has just begun to tell him about a recent success, to give a long-winded and tiresome account of his *own* successes.

How a therapist views this behavior depends on his or her primary pictures. If one of your primary pictures is the "character-defects, developmental-deficits" picture, you might attribute Jim's behavior to character defects such as:

His hair-trigger competitiveness and envy.
An inability to tolerate hearing about someone else's successes.
His inability to share the spotlight.
And, in general, his narcissism.

And I would agree that Jim is narcissistic—particularly since I am the friend Jim interrupts. Since the "character-defects, developmental-deficits" picture is only a secondary picture for me, however, I would quickly replace it with one of my four primary pictures.

Adopting the "need-to-get-something-across" primary picture, I would focus on how Jim's symptomatic behavior—his interrupting me and his inability to share the spotlight—is a consequence of his inability to get something important across. And I would try to figure out what this "something important" is. Here is what I would guess Jim would say, if he were able to figure out and say what he is unable to get across:

When you talk about a success like that, I feel envious—I have the urge to rush in and grab the spotlight from you and tell you about all of my successes.

And now we can see that Jim's problem, ironically, is that he is *not good* at being narcissistic. If he *were* good at it, he would be able to confide in me about his narcissistic sensitivities rather than be caught up in a strained, overblown, and compulsive recital of his successes. In so doing, he would be recruiting me as a resource in dealing with these sensitivities.

What Jim wants, of course, is to win my admiration. Instead, he is talking in a way that bores me, fosters my disrespect, and convinces me that he is a blowhard. He *would* win my admiration were he to make the statement that I have imagined for him—that is, were he to confide in me about his narcissistic sensitivities. I would be impressed by such a straightforward statement. I would think that he *is* special.

What I hope this example suggests is that "narcissism"—what everyone commonly thinks of as "narcissism"—is actually inept narcissism. It is inhibited, ineffectual, unsuccessful, unskillful narcissism. The term "narcissistic" has been pre-empted to mean "inept narcissism," referring as it does to people who put us off, offend us, and behave in ways that lead us to disrespect rather than admire them. We do not have a word for successful narcissism—that is, for people who effectively co-opt the spotlight, engage our interest, and win our admiration. We do not think of such people as "narcissistic." We simply think of them as interesting, admirable, and special.

But what makes Jim inept at being narcissistic? Why is he unable to confide in me about his narcissistic sensitivities? He is ashamed of them. He feels uncomfortable with them. He feels *unentitled* to them. He thinks there is something wrong with him for having these sensitivities. Here is my point: Behavior that gives the impression that the person feels *overly* entitled is typically the consequence of feeling *un*entitled.

A therapist such as Eberheart who adopts the "serves-an-unconscious-purpose" primary picture would find it unimportant that "narcissism" is really "inept narcissism." She would focus on the regressive gratification she sees the client as getting, rather than on what the client is not getting (and the difficult position from which the client is working). From such a perspective, it would be easy for Eberheart to conclude that Jim's problem is a feeling of entitlement.

A therapist like myself who adopts the "victim," "unable-to-get-something-across," and "platform-and-joint-platform" primary pictures would focus on the ineptness of the client's narcissism—on what the client is not getting rather than on what he or she *is* getting:

> Adopting the "victim" primary picture, I would focus on how hearing about someone else's success is experienced by Jim as a narcissistic assault, which he deals with by engaging in a narcissistic display.
> Adopting the "people-become-symptomatic-if-unable-to-get-something-across" primary picture, I would attribute Jim's narcissistic behavior to his inability to get across what he needs to and, in particular, to his inability to confide in me (or even in himself) about his narcissistic sensitivities.
> Adopting the "platform-and-joint-platform" primary picture, I would attribute Jim's narcissistic behavior to his inability to establish a platform (or, with me, a joint platform) from which to look at his sensitivities.

Focusing on how "narcissism" is really "inept narcissism," I would trace Jim's apparent feeling of entitlement to an underlying feeling of *un*entitlement, and, in particular, to his feeling of unentitlement to (i.e., discomfort with, sense of shame about, inability to confide in himself or others about) his narcissistic sensitivities.

A Final Factor

So those are 13 factors involved in being on the platform. And here is one more:

14. Being on the platform means being able to apply the idea of the platform to the platform itself. It means having a platform from which to monitor whether or not you are on the platform. It means having a nonanxious and non-self-accusing vantage point from which to notice that you are *not* able to do the other 13 things on this list.

How Having These Four Primary Pictures Affects My Therapeutic Work

All therapists have theories. In their actual clinical work, however, they do not always stick to them. That is where "pictures" comes in. "Pictures" are the theories that therapists *do* stick to in their clinical work (whether or not they know it and whether or not they can identify them):

> Pictures are the theories that therapists have in their minds while they listen to their clients.
> Pictures are the theories that determine what the therapist says or does at any given moment in a therapy session.

Pictures are the theories that therapists really use (except for rejected pictures, which are the theories that they specifically do *not* use, or try not to use). It is these primary, secondary, and rejected pictures that give a therapist's clinical work its special character. Here is how my primary pictures give my clinical work its special character:

1. *The "need-to-get-something-across" picture.* Focusing as I do on how clients' symptomatic responses are the result of their inability to get something across makes me a different therapist than I would be were I to focus instead on how these responses indicate developmental deficits, displacements from childhood, unconscious motives, skills deficits, unrealistic expectations, and so on.

2. *The "hidden-validity" picture.* Focusing as I do on what is valid in client's responses makes me a different therapist than I would be were I to focus on what is *in*valid in their responses.

3. *The "victim-and-joint-victims" picture.* Focusing as I do on what clients (partners) are *not* getting (how they are deprived and trapped) makes me a different therapist than I would be were I to focus on what they *are* getting (how they are being gratified, enjoying secondary gain, fulfilling primitive fantasies or unconscious purposes, getting too much from their symptoms to be willing to give them up).

4. *The "platform-and-joint-platform" picture.* Focusing as I do on enabling clients to "have" their problems makes me a different therapist than I would be were I to focus primarily on helping them eliminate these problems.

Adopting primary pictures, shifting at times into secondary pictures, and avoiding rejected pictures, is what "doing psychotherapy" *is.*

CHAPTER 28

What Happens to Marie, Paul, and the Skeptic?

If Marie and Paul Were to Adopt My Pictures

Is Marie and Paul's story going to have a happy ending?

My ultimate goal is to get my clients to adopt my four primary pictures. Let us go back in time and imagine how Marie and Paul's evening might proceed if they were already making use of them. As you remember, when Marie burst into the living room with "You never talk to me any more," Paul says:

> What have I done now? I've been sitting here bothering nobody, relaxing after a hard day, just wanting some peace and quiet. What's the big problem?

Now let us imagine that Paul has already been using my four primary pictures. That means that as soon as he has a chance to collect himself—which may be in a moment, an hour, or a week—he snaps into:

> The "need-to-get-something-across" picture, in which he recognizes that the problem is his and Marie's inability to get across their respective leading-edge feelings: "I didn't like Marie jumping down my throat with her 'You never talk to me any more.' But of course she probably said it because she wasn't able to tell me something less inflammatory earlier."
>
> Or the "hidden-validity" picture, in which he notices what is valid in Marie's responses: "Marie attacked me, so of course I defended myself. I told her how her complaint was totally illegitimate. But now that I'm not on the spot, let me try to see how it *might* be

legitimate. I've been preoccupied lately—and, so, yes, it's true, I haven't been talking to her as much as I usually do."

Or the "joint-victims" picture, in which he appreciates how Marie is stuck in something herself and is not simply trying to control him: "Marie attacked me—I'm the victim. But Marie is clearly hurting too. She had this important thing she wanted to tell me, and, of course, as soon as I felt attacked, I stopped listening."

Paul is now looking at things from Marie's point of view, as well as from his own. He is seeing her position as credible. He is sympathizing with her. He is recognizing that she has her own difficult situation to deal with and is not simply out to get him.

Since he is looking at things from Marie's point of view, Paul now has something to say that is not provocative. Shifting to his "joint-platform" picture, he tells himself:

Of course, now that I've figured all this out, I have a way to talk to Marie about what happened that isn't just blaming her for it.

We are not used to Paul's—or anyone's—being able to think in such a clear and productive way. That is my point: We are not used to people's using my four primary pictures. If they did, they would have the "instincts" they need—the easily triggered primary pictures—to deal with problems that arise in their lives and in their relationships.

So Paul goes to Marie and says:

I got angry earlier when you said I don't talk. But I've been thinking about it, and I realize that you're right: Things have been bothering me at work lately, and for some reason I haven't been telling you about it. I've shut down.

Marie is likely to be grateful to Paul for saying this. On the other hand, it may simply increase her awareness of how angry she really is:

It's not just *lately*. I can hardly remember what it feels like to have a husband who talks.

To which the old Paul would be likely to respond, "I'd say a lot more if you didn't nag me all the time." And the fight would resume. The old Paul would snap back into the "feeling-attacked, defending-myself, counterattacking, Marie-is-a-piranha" state of mind.

But remember, this is the new Paul who has adopted my four primary pictures. And one of these four is the "platform-and-joint-platform" picture. As Paul comes into the house and says to Marie, "You're right, I've haven't been talking as much lately," he is on the platform. And by that I mean:

> He has bumped himself up a level—he is thinking about the situation at the same time as he engages in it.
>
> He is a one-person consciousness-raising group (a confidant to himself) in dealing with whatever problems arise in this interaction with Marie.
>
> He is having an ongoing conversation with himself about this interaction with Marie.
>
> He is anticipating how Marie might respond and is making contingency plans.
>
> He is able to think.

Paul says to himself:

> Marie is probably going to be grateful that I'm finally seeing things from her point of view. Of course, it's possible that she *won't* be grateful—in fact, she might take advantage of my admission to press her point. So I'd better be prepared for that.

And it's good that Paul does prepare, because that is what happens: As I have just said, Marie responds to Paul's "I've been shut down lately" by saying, "It's not just *lately*. I can hardly remember what it feels like to have a husband who talks."

If Paul had not prepared himself for such a comment, he would instinctively respond, as I note above, "I'd say a lot more if you didn't nag me all the time." Since he is prepared—in fact, he has already half thought of a comeback—he is able to come out with the following tongue-in-cheek, more satisfying response:

> You're not *supposed* to say that. You're supposed to say, "I *appreciate* your admitting that you've shut down." You're supposed to say, "I already feel much better; I feel you're really listening to me." You're supposed to say, "I feel loved, you're a wonderful husband, and I'm so lucky to be married to you."

Paul is responding to Marie's angry comment with humor—which is risky. He is saying in a joking way what he *wishes* she had said. The risk is that Marie will not take it as a joke, but, instead, as his chiding her.

Fortunately for Paul, he is on the platform—which means that he is having an ongoing conversation with himself in which he can prepare for the possibility that Marie will take his comment as a putdown:

PAUL (*to himself*): If I'm lucky, Marie will laugh and it'll break the tension. It'll turn things around. But it's possible that she won't take it as a joke. So I'd better prepare for that.

MARIE (*to Paul*): Well, I *don't* feel better. I don't *care* that you're listening *now*—I needed you to listen *before*. And I don't feel any of those other fantasies of yours, either. What I *do* feel is unlucky to be married to you.

Had Paul not prepared for this verbal slap, he might instinctively respond, "Well, I feel unlucky to be married to you, too." But since he has prepared, he is able to let it go for the moment and then, later in the evening, after Marie has had a chance to cool down, to go to her and say:

PAUL: Do you really feel, as you were saying earlier, that I haven't been talking *or* listening for a long, long time—that I've abandoned you?

MARIE (*sighs in relief*): Yes.

Here Paul is using another of my primary pictures: the "need-to-get-something-across" picture. Snapping into this picture, Paul tries to figure out what Marie is suffering from being unable to get across. And immediately it becomes obvious, since it is exactly what she has been saying: She feels he has been shut down for a long time. Paul has created a *joint* platform from which he and Marie can look nonangrily and nondefensively at her complaint.

So that is an example of how it might look if Paul were to adopt my four primary pictures. But let us suppose that it is *Marie* who does so, and let us go back in time and reconstruct the fight from this point of view. Immediately after bursting into the living room and telling Paul, "You never talk to me any more," she has the following "from-the-platform" conversation with herself:

Wow, where did that come from?
I didn't know I was that angry.
Paul is going to be shocked—*I'm* shocked.
He's going to get defensive.
So I'd better get ready for it.
And that's going to be hard, because I hate it when Paul gets defensive.
So I'd better prepare to hate it.
Of course, I could try to smooth things over.

I could say, "Wow, where did that come from? I didn't know I was
that angry."
Paul wouldn't get defensive then.
So that's what I should do.
But I don't feel like doing it.
I've been smoothing things over my whole life.
I'm going to let the chips fall where they may.
Okay, Paul. Give me your best shot.

And Paul gives her his best shot:

What have I done now? I've been sitting here bothering nobody,
relaxing after a hard day, just wanting some peace and quiet.
What's the big problem?

Here is the "from-the-platform" conversation that Marie has with
herself:

So *that's* his best shot.
It's a pretty good one—not fatal, but a definite ouch.
I hate it when Paul goes into his "Who, me? I'm an innocent
bystander" number.
Of course, *he* hates it when I accuse him of not talking. So maybe
we're even. (Here Marie has momentarily snapped into the "we're-
both-feeling-frustrated-by-the-other, we're-joint-victims" primary
picture.)
I could straighten it out right now. I could *admit* that my "You never
talk to me any more" was an attack. Paul would appreciate that.
(And here she has snapped into the "what-does-Paul-need-me-to-
appreciate? what-does-he-need-to-get-across-to-me-to-stop-being-
symptomatic?" primary picture.)
And then I could say, "And I'm sorry I attacked you, because there
was something important I wanted to say, and attacking you is a
pretty dumb way to get you to listen."
Unless he is *really* angry, Paul would appreciate my saying that—in
which case, he might then be able to listen.
So that would be the *smart* thing for me to do.
But I don't feel like doing it.
Being smart isn't worth it if it means smoothing the way yet again.
What I feel like doing is blasting Paul for his "Who-me? I-was-just-
sitting-here-when-you-came-in-like-the-Terminator" routine.
And I know exactly how to do it.

Marie says to Paul:

Don't act so surprised. You know *exactly* what I'm talking about.

Being on the platform does not necessarily mean that Marie has to say anything different than she would if she were not on the platform. (In fact, so far Marie is saying exactly what I have described her as saying in Chapter 11.) What is crucial is that Marie is *thinking* in a different way. And thinking differently will ultimately lead to her behaving differently.

For the next several exchanges, however, the argument continues as I have described in Chapter 11:

MARIE: You never talk to me—not even tonight, when I really needed it.
PAUL: Why didn't you tell me you wanted to talk? I'm not a mind reader.
MARIE: How could you possibly *not* know? I told you how everything
        went wrong today.
PAUL: What about Wednesday, when you were upset about your mother
        and we spent the whole evening—

Here is the "from-the-platform" conversation that Marie has with herself at this point:

This fight is getting ridiculous.
I want to end it now.
But I have such a great comeback that I can't resist.

So she continues:

MARIE: I remember it well. You said, "Oh, that's too bad," and spent the
        whole evening watching television.
PAUL: You were with people all day today. I thought you wanted time to
        yourself.

Here is Marie's next "from-the-platform" conversation with herself:

It wasn't as great a comeback as I'd thought.
He was able to answer it.
Not a terrific answer—but it was an answer.
Paul is spunky today.
I'm sick of this.
Enough of my comebacks.
Time to end the fight.

She says to Paul:

This isn't how I wanted the evening to go. I wanted things to be better between us.

And she has this "from-the-platform" conversation with herself:

Oh-oh, Paul might hear that as blaming—that I'm suggesting it's because of *him* that things haven't gone right.
I can fix that.

To Paul, she continues:

Of course, how nice can things be if I'm going to break into the living room and accuse you of never talking to me any more?

And to *herself* she continues:

That should fix it.
Paul can't possibly feel blamed now.
But, oh-oh. I know what he's going to do.
He's going to answer my "Of course, how nice can things be if I'm going to break into the living room and accuse you of never talking to me any more?" with "That's right. Why do you always have to attack me?"
He's going to take advantage of my admission to rub it in.
I just *know* he's going to do that.
I wish I hadn't set him up like that.

And Paul says just what she fears:

That's right. Why do you always have to attack me?

Here is Marie's next "from-the-platform" conversation with herself:

I can't stand it.
I thought I was prepared for it, but there's no way to prepare for it.
It presses all my buttons.
I know I should let it go. It's not going to help either of us if I strike back.
It'll just make things worse.
But I just don't care.

She tells Paul:

When I *don't* attack—when I say things in a nice way—you don't
listen then either.

Marie's "from-the-platform" conversation with herself:

I was mistaken—it *did* help one of us. It helped *me*. I feel better for
having said it. It was worth it.
Even if there's a price to pay.

Paul replies:

When have you ever, even once, said things in a nice way?

Marie says to herself, from the platform:

There's the price.
It's not too bad a price—I can afford it.
I could argue with him—I could insist that I do say things in a nice
way sometimes . . . often.
But that would just continue the fight.
So I'll accept what he said.
That'll surprise him.
And it might end the fight.

MARIE (*to Paul*): Well, let me *try* to say this differently then. Instead of
"You never talk to me any more," I could say, "You know, a long
time ago, when we first met, it seemed that we had endless things
to say to each other. And I miss it."
PAUL: Yes, I know what you mean; I miss it too.

Here is the "from-the-platform" conversation that Marie has with
herself:

Well, that worked out well.
And it felt good.
I said what I had to say, and in a way that wasn't an attack.
And Paul was able to listen to me.
But did I lose something in the translation? What happened to the
attack?
Did I suppress it?

> Did I revert to my old habit of smoothing things over?
> I don't think so—but I'm not sure.
> I'll have to keep my eyes open. If I *did* suppress my anger, it'll pop up—and then I'll know.

So that is how things might go if *Marie* were to adopt my four primary pictures—just as earlier I have shown what might happen if Paul were to adopt them.

Things would go even better, of course, if *both* Marie and Paul were to adopt these pictures. They would be able to create a permanent joint platform—an ongoing shared vantage point—from which to monitor their relationship.

This is what a happy ending would look like—not "They lived happily ever after," but rather "They kept their wits about them when they were *un*happy." It is a happy ending that illustrates my therapeutic goal, which is to get clients to adopt my four primary pictures.

Four Types of Client Responses

I have found, however, that it is often hard to get clients to adopt my pictures. When I sat down to try to figure out more about it, I was able to identify four types of client responses.

Client Type 1: Those Who Are Already on the Verge of Adopting My Four Primary Pictures

Type 1 clients are those who do not require much to get them to adopt one or more of my pictures. They get the idea, and they like the idea.

Let us say that in attempting to promote the "platform-and-joint-platform" primary picture for Marie and Paul, I make up several conversations for them in which, instead of anxiously seeking immediate solutions (which is what they usually do), I have them calmly acknowledge the lack of an immediate solution. I tell them:

> Okay, so at this point in the conversation I'm making up, Paul, you'd say to Marie, "I guess this is one of those times that we don't have an immediate solution." And Marie, you'd say, "I guess you're right."

Marie and Paul come back the next week and say:

MARIE (*to therapist*): We were talking about the problem of our different needs for talking, and it did help to realize that we don't have to solve every problem right away.

PAUL: It takes the pressure off.

MARIE: We can do what you did last week and just recognize that we don't have an immediate solution.

All it takes for Marie and Paul to adopt this "from-the-platform, not-anxiously-having-to-solve-the-problem-right-away" perspective is a little push. Of course, they do *need* the push. Without it, they could be on the verge of getting it, but not quite getting it, for the rest of their lives.

Client Type 2: Those for Whom My Primary Pictures Are Their Rejected Pictures

Type 2 clients are those who, unlike Type 1 clients, do not find the ideas implicit in my four primary pictures helpful and relieving:

> *Regarding the "hidden-validity" primary picture*, these clients are mystified by my effort to reveal the validity in their responses. They cannot understand why I don't agree with them that their responses are inappropriate, unacceptable, and unforgivable.
>
> *Regarding the "need-to-get-something-across" primary picture*, these clients are mystified by my effort to demonstrate that what they see as their immature and irrational behavior is the result of feeling unentitled to ordinary adult feelings. They cannot understand why I don't agree with them that their problem is simply that they are immature and irrational—or, at least, that their partners are.
>
> *Regarding the "victim-and-joint-victims" primary picture*, these clients are mystified by my effort to show them that they are victims. "It's my own fault," such a client says in effect; "I'm doing it to myself."
>
> *Regarding the "platform-and-joint-platform" primary picture*, these clients are mystified by my effort to show that the problem is their "inability to have the problem"—that is, their anxious need to solve it right away. They cannot understand why I don't agree with them that they should be able to do away with the problem immediately. They are also mystified by my accepting problems as inevitable and my emphasis on developing a platform from which to talk about them. They cannot understand why I don't agree with them that they should not be having problems in the first place.

Such clients often feel that I am letting them off too easy, pulling my punches, holding back what I really think, being the nice guy. They think I am not doing my job, which they see as:

Telling them what they are doing wrong.
Setting them straight.
Giving them the kick in the pants they think they need.

These clients are committed to a way of thinking that I see as the problem. Of course, from their point of view, I am committed to a way of thinking that *they* see as the problem.

So what do I do? The same thing I do with partners who are in conflict with each other. Just as I try to create a joint platform from which partners can talk about their conflict, I try to create a joint platform from which the client (or partners) and I can talk about *our* conflict (i.e., our contrasting views), and the following in particular:

How they feel thrown off by me.
How they feel I am failing to appreciate the problem.
How they feel mystified and frustrated by my not doing what they
    believe is necessary to solve their problems—namely, telling them
    what they are doing wrong and telling them how to do it right.
How, as I see it, they are already telling themselves what they are
    doing wrong (and kicking themselves in the pants)—and that is
    the problem.
How they are in the difficult position of having a therapist they feel
    does not understand them.

So what happens? Sometimes I get these clients to accept my view; that is, they do begin to develop a sense of the usefulness of my four primary pictures. Sometimes they get me to accept their view; that is, they show me how they *do* profit from being told what to do or from a kick in the pants. Sometimes they transfer to another therapist who is more in agreement with their approach to things.

But no matter what happens, I try to create a platform from which we can talk about it.

Client Type 3: Those for Whom My Primary Pictures Are Weak Secondary Pictures

Type 3 clients are those who, unlike Type 2 clients, do get something from my demonstrations of my four pictures. But the ideas do not stick.

Minutes—or even seconds—later, they return to their usual way of thinking:

> Looking at what is invalid in their own and/or their partners'
> responses, rather than looking at what is valid.
>
> Viewing their (or their partners') provocative behavior as the con-
> sequences of childish impulses, rather than as an inability to get
> across ordinary adult feelings.
>
> Seeing themselves (or themselves and their partners) as uncon-
> sciously wanting their problems because they are getting some-
> thing from them, rather than as stuck in something they don't
> want and thus as joint victims.
>
> Solving problems, rather than creating a platform (or joint platform)
> from which to look at them.

These clients return to their usual modes of thinking so quickly that
I am not certain whether they have adopted my way of thinking even
for that moment.

How do I deal with this? I try to establish a platform from which
we can discuss the contrast between their modes of thinking and my
modes of thinking.

Client Type 4: Those for Whom My Primary Pictures Are Clear Secondary Pictures

Type 4 clients are those who, unlike Type 3 clients, do clearly adopt my
four primary pictures. They respond to my discussions or demonstrations of the pictures by adopting them as firm secondary pictures. They
adopt them for more than a moment—often, in fact, for the remainder
of the session, or even longer. These clients, however, typically return
for the following session having completely forgotten the pictures. My
goal is to make these secondary pictures more a part of their everyday
lives—and, ultimately, to turn them into primary pictures.

My task with all four types of client responses is:

> To construct a platform from which my clients can look at their
> various primary, secondary, and rejected pictures.
>
> To construct a joint platform from which they and I can talk about
> our shared and unshared pictures.

Final Dialogue between the Author and the Skeptic

Wile (*to Skeptic*): So that's my book. What do you think of it?

Skeptic: I think you've got a big problem.

Wile: Oh?

Skeptic: Some of your readers are going to come away thinking that it's *easy* to adopt your four pictures. When they find out that it isn't, they're going to get discouraged.

Wile: And the other readers?

Skeptic: They're going to come away thinking that it's too *hard* to adopt your four pictures. They're going to donate your book to the recycling bin.

Wile: Oh-oh. How do you know all this?

Skeptic: Because I've been going back and forth between those two reactions myself.

Wile: Well, maybe I shouldn't have published it then.

Skeptic: Wait a minute! Where's your "sitting with the problem"? Where's your "not anxiously having to solve it right away"? I just mention that your book has some problems, and what do you do? You immediately conclude that you shouldn't publish it. Where's the platform? Do I have to remind you of your own theory?

Wile: Well, yes, you might have to—because it's easy to forget—even if it *is* my theory. And, if I may say so, you seem to be developing a sense for it.

Skeptic (*skeptically*): You think so, huh?

Wile: I do. And you've just shown how people can help one another create a platform.

Skeptic: Well, okay, but I still think it's a problem when the guy who invented the idea of the platform goes around falling off it.

Wile: That's why I rely on creating a platform for noticing how I slip on and off the platform. And it looks as if I can count on you to help.

Closing Comment

So that is the view of relationships and the theory of therapy that emerge from this look at Marie and Paul's evening. I have tried:

> To convince you of the value of my four primary pictures, or, if not, at least to get you thinking about your own pictures.
>
> To promote the view of life as a sequence of states of mind—and

pictures—and to show how, while the client is going through his or her own states of mind and pictures, so is the therapist.

To show that everyone's main problem—feeling unentitled to feelings—is ultimately unsolvable, which is where the platform comes in. The platform is the premier way to deal with unsolvable problems.

I hope that reading about this evening in the life of Marie and Paul will change all your nights—and all your days—or, better yet, will help you develop a platform from which to notice whether and in what ways they do change.

References

American Psychiatric Association. (1987). *Diagnostic and statistical manual of mental disorders* (3rd ed., rev.) Washington, DC: Author.

Apfelbaum, B. (1966). On ego psychology: A critique of the structural approach to psychoanalysis. *International Journal of Psycho-Analysis, 47,* 451–475.

Apfelbaum, B. (1977). A contribution to the development of the behavioral-analytic sex therapy model. *Journal of Sex and Marital Therapy, 3,* 128–138.

Apfelbaum, B. (1982a, Spring). Letter to the editor. *The California State Psychologist,* p. 16.

Apfelbaum, B. (1982b). The clinical necessity for Kohut's self theory. *Voices, 18,* 43–49.

Apfelbaum, B. (1983). Introduction. In B. Apfelbaum (Chair), *Ego analysis and ego psychology.* Symposium conducted at the meeting of the American Psychological Association, Anaheim, CA.

Apfelbaum, B. (1988). An ego-analytic perspective on desire disorders. In S. Leiblum & L. Rosen (Eds.), *Sexual desire disorders* (pp. 75–104). New York: Guilford Press.

Apfelbaum, B., & Apfelbaum, C. (1985). The ego-analytic approach to sexual apathy. In D. C. Goldberg (Ed.), *Contemporary marriage: Special issues in couples therapy* (pp. 439–481). Homewood, IL: Dorsey Press.

Apfelbaum, B., & Gill, M. M. (1989). Ego analysis and the relativity of defense: Technical implications of the structural theory. *Journal of the American Psychoanalytic Association, 37,* 1071–1096.

Beneke, T. (1988, October 7). A conversation with dissident Freud scholar Jeffrey Masson. *Express* (Berkeley), pp. 1, 10–15.

Christensen, A., Jacobson, N. S., & Babcock, J. C. (in press). Integrative behavioral couple therapy. In N. S. Jacobson & A. S. Gurman (Eds.), *Clinical handbook of marital therapy* (2nd ed.). New York: Guilford Press.

Faber, A., & Mazlish, E. (1975). *Liberated parents/liberated children.* New York: Avon. (Original work published 1974)

Faber, A., & Mazlish, E. (1982). *How to talk so kids will listen and listen so kids will talk.* New York: Avon. (Original work published 1980)

Fenichel, O. (1941). *Problems of psychoanalytic technique.* New York: Psychoanalytic Quarterly.

Freud, S. (1959). Inhibitions, symptoms and anxiety. In J. Strachey (Ed. and Trans.), *The standard edition of the complete psychological works of Sigmund Freud* (Vol. 20, pp. 77–174). London: Hogarth Press. (Original work published 1926)

Freud, S. (1960). The psychopathology of everyday life. In J. Strachey (Ed. and Trans.), *The standard edition of the complete psychological works of Sigmund Freud* (Vol. 6). London: Hogarth Press. (Original work published 1901)

Gray, P. (1982). "Developmental lag" in the evolution of technique for psychoanalysis of neurotic conflict. *Journal of the American Psychoanalytic Association, 30*, 621–655.

Horowitz, M. J. (1987). States of mind: configurational analysis of individual psychology (2nd ed.). New York: Plenum.

Jacobson, N. S., & Holtzworth-Munroe, A. (1986). Marital therapy: A social learning–cognitive perspective. In N. S. Jacobson & A. S. Gurman (Eds.), *Clinical handbook of marital therapy* (pp. 22–70). New York: Guilford Press.

Kohut, H. (1984). *How does analysis cure?* Chicago: University of Chicago Press.

Meichenbaum, D. (1991, May 23–24). *Cognitive-behavioral psychotherapy: Focus on treatment of affective disorders.* Workshop sponsored by the Institute for the Advancement of Human Behavior, San Diego.

Ornstein, R. (1989). *Multimind.* New York: Anchor Books (Doubleday).

Simon, R. (1992). Like a friendly editor: An interview with Lynn Hoffman. In R. Simon, *One on one: Conversations with the shapers of family therapy* (pp. 159–165). Washington, DC: *The Family Therapy Networker*/New York: Guilford Press.

Wachtel, P. L. (1977). *Psychoanalysis and behavior therapy: Toward an integration.* New York: Basic Books.

Wachtel, P. L. (1993). *Therapeutic communication: Principles and effective practice.* New York: Guilford Press.

Wile, D. B. (1981). *Couples therapy: A nontraditional approach.* New York: Wiley.

Wile, D. B. (1984). Kohut, Kernberg, and accusatory interpretations. *Psychotherapy: Theory, Research, Practice, and Training, 21*(3), 353–364.

Wile, D. B. (1985a). Psychotherapy by precedent: Unexamined legacies from pre-1920 psychoanalysis. *Psychotherapy: Theory, Research, Practice, and Training, 22*(4), 793–802.

Wile, D. B. (1985b). Phases of relationship development. In D.C. Goldberg (Ed.), *Contemporary marriage: Special issues in couples therapy* (pp. 35–61). Homewood, IL: Dorsey Press.

Wile, D. B. (1987). An even more offensive theory. In W. Dryden (Ed.), *Key cases in psychotherapy* (pp. 78–102). London: Croom Helm.

Wile, D. B. (1988). *After the honeymoon: How conflict can improve your relationship.* New York: Wiley.

Wile, D. B. (in press-a). The ego-analytic approach to emotion in couples therapy. In S. M. Johnson & L. S. Greenberg (Eds.), *The heart of the matter: Perspectives on emotion in marital therapy.* New York: Brunner/Mazel.

Wile, D. B. (in press-b). The ego-analytic approach to couples therapy. In N. S. Jacobson & A. S. Gurman (Eds.), *The clinical handbook of couple therapy* (2nd ed.). New York: Guilford Press.

Index